BROKEN TO BREATHFUL

*Simple Breathwork and Daily Rituals
For Emotional Healing, Resilience and
Nervous System Regulation*

Romy Krakauer Limenes

Copyright © 2025 Romy Krakauer Limenes

Published by A Tree Fell On Me

All rights reserved. No part of this book may be reproduced, stored in a retrieval system, or transmitted in any form or by any means—electronic, mechanical, photocopying, recording, or otherwise—without the prior written permission of the author or publisher, except in the case of brief quotations embodied in critical articles or reviews.

This book is for personal use only. You may not sell, distribute, paraphrase, quote, or modify any part of its contents without express written consent from the author or publisher.

Disclaimer

The contents of this book are intended for educational and inspirational purposes only. While every effort has been made to present accurate, up-to-date, and reliable information, no guarantees or warranties are made, either express or implied. The author does not dispense legal, financial, or medical advice. The practices shared here reflect personal experience and are not a substitute for professional care. Always consult a qualified practitioner before beginning any healing, breathwork, or therapeutic practice.

By reading this book, you agree that the author and publisher are not liable for any damages, losses, or injuries, direct or indirect, that may occur as a result of the application or interpretation of the information herein.

Memoir & Creative Nonfiction Disclosure

This book is a work of creative nonfiction and memoir. It reflects the author's true experiences, emotions, and recollections to the best of her ability. Names, locations, and identifying details have been changed or omitted to protect the privacy of individuals. Any resemblance to real people, living or dead, is purely coincidental unless otherwise stated.

The intention in sharing this story is not to defame or harm, but to bear witness, reclaim voice, and contribute to healing—personal and collective. It is offered in good faith, with care, clarity, and respect.

EPIGRAPH

"When we speak we are afraid our words will not be heard or welcomed. But when we are silent, we are still afraid. So it is better to speak."

— Audre Lorde

DEDICATION

To Emil and Lucy—
You are my heart.
Your laughter and love bring me home, again and again.
I love you beyond words.

To Natasha—
Your steady presence has been a gift.
Thank you for walking beside me with kindness,
humor, and unwavering care.
You are the sister my soul has always known.

TABLE OF CONTENTS

INTRODUCTION 1

PART ONE | THE STORM: THE BREAKING POINT THAT BECAME THE BEGINNING 5

CHAPTER 1 | UPENDED 7

CHAPTER 2 | JAIL 10

CHAPTER 3 | FREEDOM? 15

CHAPTER 4 | UNFATHOMABLE 21

CHAPTER 5 | A NEW FIGHT 28

PART TWO | BRIDGE AND ANCHOR: BREATHING WITH ATTENTION AND INTENTION 30

CHAPTER 6 | THE WISDOM OF REGULATION 32

CHAPTER 7 | THE RITUAL OF RETURN 37

CHAPTER 8 | THE ALCHEMY OF EMOTION 43

PART THREE | THE LIFELINES: THREADS OF RETURN AND REMEMBRANCE 49

CHAPTER 9 | RADICAL SELF-LOVE—YOU ARE ENOUGH 52

CHAPTER 10 | FEEL ALL YOUR FEELINGS—THEY ARE MEANT TO BE FELT 58

CHAPTER 11 | BEND—MOVE YOUR BODY AND LET IT MOVE YOU 64

CHAPTER 12 | BREATHE—COME BACK TO YOUR SENSES 68

CHAPTER 13 | SOUND—LISTEN DEEPLY, EXPRESS FREELY 72

CHAPTER 14 | CIRCLE—BE HELD, HOLD OTHERS 76

CHAPTER 15 | EXPRESS—LET YOUR TRUTH BE SEEN 81

CHAPTER 16 | HEART & HANDS—SERVICE, GRATITUDE, AND TRUST 85

CHAPTER 17 | BODY TEMPLE—CARE FOR THE VESSEL THAT CARRIES YOU 90

PART FOUR | FROM AIR TO EMBODIMENT: A GUIDE TO BREATHWORK PRACTICES 96

CHAPTER 18 | BREATHING WITH ATTENTION 103

CHAPTER 19 | BREATHING WITH INTENTION 108

CHAPTER 20 | MORE MEDICINE 114

CHAPTER 21 | BREATHING FOR EMOTIONAL RELEASE 120

INTEGRATION | THE BREATH WITHIN AND THROUGHOUT 126

CONCLUSION | COMING HOME 127

EPILOGUE | A FINAL NOTE ON SOVEREIGNTY (AND WHAT COMES NEXT) 131

AFTERWORD | A CALL FOR CHANGE 134

STAY CONNECTED WITH ME 137
ABOUT THE AUTHOR 138
ROMY'S FAVORITE READS 139
REFERENCES 143

INTRODUCTION

I never imagined I'd be where I am today. Like most people, I lived my life doing my best to find balance and keep moving forward. Then, in an instant, everything changed. One event shattered my sense of safety and identity, leaving me stripped of power, disoriented by injustice, and caught in a system more invested in preserving its own narrative than in seeking the truth.

And yet, in that darkness, something began to shift. What felt like an ending slowly revealed itself as a beginning. That rupture—though devastating—became a doorway. It cracked me open, not just to pain, but to a kind of healing I didn't even know I needed. Leading me to breathwork—simple, intentional breathing—and a handful of practices that grounded me and helped me make sense of what felt impossible. I came to call them the Lifelines.

These Lifelines didn't change what had happened, but they helped me find steadiness, reconnect with my body, and reclaim a sense of agency and trust in myself.

For over twenty years, I worked as a nurse—a role that asked me to show up with steadiness and deep respect for the human experience. I witnessed birth, death, and everything in between. I learned not just about the human body, but what it truly means to hold space for someone. Still, it wasn't until my own crisis that I began to understand what healing really means—not just physically, but emotionally, mentally, and spiritually.

I knew talk therapy. I had spent years unearthing and analyzing my past. But as I stumbled through this new landscape of trauma—exhausted, untethered, desperate for relief—I realized that insight alone couldn't carry me. I didn't just need to understand my pain. I needed to move through it, feel it, and transmute it.

That's when I found breathwork. At first, I was skeptical. Could something so basic—so natural—as breathing really help me navigate trauma, calm my nervous system, and reconnect with myself? I wasn't sure. But I was willing to try.

My initial experiences weren't easy. While others described immediate breakthroughs, I felt agitated, resistant, even disconnected. The main technique I would eventually teach—Conscious Connected Breath—was especially challenging. I had to go slowly, modify it to meet my nervous system where it was. At first, nothing felt like it was working.

But with patient guidance and a safe space to explore, something began to open. I started to soften. To feel. To stay. Beneath the resistance was grief, stillness, and also a quiet sense that maybe I wasn't broken after all.

Breathwork became a way to stay with myself when everything felt overwhelming. It gave me the strength to be present with the parts of me I had long avoided. It became both a resource and a refuge—a way to meet what was hard without running from it. Over time, I didn't just feel better—I began to feel whole. I began to feel myself again.

More than a coping tool, breath became a way to reclaim something essential. It reminded me: I am allowed to take up space. I am safe in my body. I don't have to earn my worth. Each breath became a quiet, powerful act of self-remembering and reclamation.

What started as a personal practice soon became a calling. I trained as a certified breathwork facilitator and trauma-informed coach—not just to deepen my own understanding, but to share with others the tools that had anchored me when everything felt unsteady.

Breathwork helped me find stable ground again. The Lifelines guided me back to myself. From here, I began to slowly rebuild from the inside out.

Part One shares the personal story behind this work—the event that cracked my life wide open and the unraveling that followed. What initially felt random and senseless revealed itself as a call to turn inward.

Part Two explores the "what" and "why"—the science, theory, and nervous system principles behind breathwork. If you're like me, you don't just want to know *how* to do something, you also want to *understand why* it works. This section lays the foundation to support the practices and principles ahead.

Parts Three and Four make it tangible. You'll find guided breathwork practices and daily Lifeline rituals—the tools I leaned on during my hardest days and still return to now. These practices are simple, adaptable, and meet you where you are. They aren't one-time fixes; they're steady supports that grow stronger with use.

You don't have to read this book straight through. Follow your instincts. Start with the memoir, or skip to the practices. Let it meet you where you are. These practices helped me reconnect with myself after everything fell apart, but they're not the only way. You may already have tools or rituals that work for you. Take what resonates. Leave what doesn't.

This book is a personal offering—a way of making meaning from my own experience and passing along something positive. It's brief by design. Sometimes, simplicity speaks the loudest.

If you're in a hard season—feeling lost, overwhelmed, or unsure where to start—let this book be a steady companion.

You don't have to navigate this alone.

PART ONE | THE STORM: THE BREAKING POINT THAT BECAME THE BEGINNING

"How many times does something have to happen to you before something occurs to you?

—Robert Frost

In the pages that follow, I'll share my story as honestly as I can—how I remember it and how it unfolded. I should say upfront: for the first seven hours of what I consider the beginning of this story, I experienced complete amnesia. Some pieces I simply cannot speak to.

What I was able to reconstruct comes from body cam footage, witness statements, public records, and the support of a private investigator and legal counsel. I've included only what feels essential to the heart of this book. Some of what I uncovered was more disturbing than what's written here—but this is not a tell-all. It's a story about healing, reclamation, and finding steadiness in the aftermath.

I am not here to sensationalize or seek vengeance. Names, locations, and identifying details are intentionally omitted. I never had the chance to tell my story in a courtroom, so this is my way of reclaiming my voice and honoring what I lived. Equally important—it is a message to anyone who has been unjustly silenced:

You are not alone.
Your voice matters.

I came to realize that my experience is not rare. Stories like mine happen every day, across every community. What makes it harder is how preventable so much of it is. Gaps in accessible testing, insufficient training for first responders, and cultural biases—especially around drug-facilitated assault—leave survivors unsupported and doubted, while the harm-doers often go unaccountable.

Some moments, though fragmented, are etched into my body. They returned not as memories, but as physical truths—flashes of sensation and instinct that no amnesia could erase.

This is where the story begins.

CHAPTER 1 | UPENDED

The fluorescent lights hum overhead, casting an artificial brightness that makes everything feel cold and sterile. I blink, trying to clear the haze clouding my vision, and immediately realize I'm not alone. Figures move around me—blurry, unfamiliar. The air smells of antiseptic and something metallic. Machines beep. Footsteps echo. Voices murmur low.

I know this place. Well.

I've worked as a nurse for over twenty years. This is my world—or at least, it was. But something is wrong. Very wrong.

My pulse quickens. Panic rises. And then I hear it:

"You fucking douchebag!"

The voice is mine. But I don't recognize it at first. My throat burns. My words are laced with rage—raw, unfiltered. I don't understand why I'm so furious. Why I'm lashing out.

I turn and see him—a man in light blue scrubs. A doctor, maybe. He's calm. Too calm. Something about him feels off.

I snap.

I rip the IV catheter from my arm. It slides out with a dull tug. I hurl it across the room. It hits the wall with a sharp crack, shattering the momentary silence.

Why am I so angry?

Then: hands. All over me. Restraining. A sting in my arm. Someone injects something.

The world spins. Everything blurs.

Then: black.

I wake, sitting on the edge of a gurney. My body is too still. Heavy. Sedated. My head is a stone. Thoughts struggle to form.

There's a man in the hallway. Watching. A "sitter."

I've seen this before—patients under observation for safety. But this time, the realization hits hard:

I'm the one being watched.

Before I can process it, three police officers enter the room. The air shifts—tight, electric. I don't even have time to speak before they close in.

One officer yanks my arms behind my back. Pain shoots through my shoulders. My wrists scream.

"You have the right to remain silent..."

The words crash into me—familiar from TV, surreal in real life. My life.

"What am I being arrested for?" I blurt. But part of me doesn't want to hear the answer.

"You threatened the victim," one officer says. His voice is smug. Final.

Victim.

The word hits harder than the cuffs cutting into my skin. I try to understand. But there's nothing. No memory. Just a void.

The clock reads just past midnight. I remember that it's Wednesday.

Fragments surface. I'd dropped my kids off at their dad's. I was going to swim, but it was too hot. I was tired.
So I decided to grab lunch instead.

They lead me down the hall. My steps are uneven. The cuffs bite into my wrists. My body aches. But nothing comes close to the shame.

We pass through the ER. Voices echo. Gurneys roll. Stale air clings to everything.

Then I notice the eyes.
Watching. Judging. Pitying.

In that moment, I'm not a nurse. Not a mother. Not a woman in need.
I'm a spectacle.

Shame wraps around me like a second skin. I lower my gaze. Try to disappear.

But I can't.

So I do the only thing I can: keep walking. One foot in front of the other.
Holding on by a thread.
Trying not to fall apart as my dignity slips quietly away.

CHAPTER 2 | JAIL

I'm led to a police SUV. The man behind the wheel isn't one of the officers who escorted me from the hospital, but it hardly matters now. As he guides me into the back seat, time slows. His motion is unexpectedly gentle—almost tender—a jarring contrast to the restraining hands from before.

The warmth inside the vehicle wraps around me like a blanket. It feels oddly safe. The hum of the engine, the sway of the ride—surreal. Disorienting.

I sit silently, numb. The officer's small talk floats around me, detached, like background noise. He could be a taxi driver or a hotel clerk. Not someone driving me to jail.

It's dizzying. I've fallen into someone else's life.

We pull into an underground garage lit by flickering fluorescent lights. Tires echo off concrete. The engine cuts. Silence.

More officers await. They move quickly, collecting my belongings with practiced indifference. My flip-flops slap against the cold ground. My cotton dress clings in the humid air.

I'm handed a pair of pants. Finally, something that makes sense. I slip them on, grateful. The fabric is soft on my bare legs.

I glance down at my sweater. It feels like a relic from another life. I'd grabbed it absentmindedly on my way out, even though the day was blistering. My dress was tight, clingy. I felt self-conscious in it anywhere but the pool, so I threw on the sweater to obscure the shape of me.

I'd planned to swim laps after dropping the kids at their dad's. But on a whim—tired, overheated—I changed course. A cold beer and a late lunch sounded better. So I drove downtown. Through familiar streets. My streets. The ones where I live, work, raise my children.

And now, I'm here. Cuffed. In jail. My life upended.

I take a shaky breath. I still don't understand how it unraveled so fast.

They lead me into a holding room—sterile, fluorescent, with bolted chairs lined up like a DMV. Not barred cells like in the movies, but somehow worse in its impersonality.

About ten others sit slouched, silent. No one looks up. Their faces are blank, resigned. A TV flickers in the background—reruns, commercials, laughing people. The contrast is cruel.

A red line stretches across the floor: "Do Not Cross This Line." It feels symbolic. A barrier I can't cross. Jail staff move freely on the other side—laughing, chatting. Their normalcy slices through me.

It's nearly 1:00 a.m.

I retrace my steps as best I can.

It was a Wednesday—early dismissal day. I'd left home around noon to pick up my daughter. She had a doctor's appointment, and afterward, we stopped at the park before grabbing a quick slice of pizza. Then I dropped her off at her dad's, where she'd stay for the next five days.

I had the evening to myself. The plan was to swim, then unwind at home with some Netflix.

But I was tired. Hungry.

On an impulse, I skipped the pool and went for a late lunch instead.

That's all it took. One decision. One shift.

Then comes the gut punch: Mimi.

My rescue dog. My companion. Sensitive. Anxious. She's never been without me this long. Over twelve hours now. She must be pacing, confused, waiting. The thought guts me. I curl with guilt and helplessness.

I try to pull myself together. I call out—careful not to cross the red line.

"Excuse me… how long will I be here? When will I find out what's going on?"

The officers respond politely, but with distance. I'm told I can't be released until the victim is notified. The charge is classified as violent.

Victim.

The word sends a fresh wave of nausea through my body. I can't fathom it. Could I have hurt someone? I don't remember. I can't remember. The thought is unbearable.

The AC blasts nonstop. I shiver, shrinking into myself. Everyone is cold. No blankets. No jackets. Just thin clothing and freezing air.

A woman nearby tucks her arms into her t-shirt. Her eyes are glazed. Another stumbles from the bathroom, retching, collapsing, then doing it again. No one reacts. Pain is background noise here.

I wish I could do something to help. But I can't even keep myself warm.

Time drips. Hours crawl. The cold digs deep.

I spot the pay phones—lined up against the wall in the same crowded room. There's no privacy. The thought of making a call, of trying to figure out how I'm going to get bailed out, is humiliating. I don't have my glasses, and my eyes are so swollen it takes me several tries just to dial the number for a bail bondsman.

A voice answers.

I explain, stumbling through it. The bail is $100,000. I need $10,000 to get out.

The number stuns me. Then: relief. I think of my savings. I can cover it. I never imagined needing that money for this. But I'm grateful now.

The bail bondsman is kind. Calm. He says the process has started. I'll be out soon. Otherwise, I'd have to wait five days for court due to the holiday weekend.

Five days?!

I can't even fathom it. I quickly push the thought away.

My face throbs.

There are no mirrors, but I can feel the damage. The swelling. The bruises. Pain maps my skin.

A woman approaches.

"What happened to your face? It looks really bad."

Her voice is blunt, not cruel. I flinch under her gaze. Her words land harder than the bruises.

"The officers… said I assaulted someone," I whisper. "Then I fell. That's how I got hurt. I can't remember anything."

I pause. "I've never hurt anyone before."

She studies me. Curiosity, maybe pity. I can't tell. I don't know what to feel. I'm unraveling. Barely holding on.

This isn't who I am.

I'm the caregiver. The nurse. The helper.

Not this.
Not here.

But this is happening.
I am here.
And I have to find a way through.

CHAPTER 3 | FREEDOM?

After what feels like an eternity, I'm finally released. Eleven hours of waiting, suppressing panic, sitting in confusion—and now, I'm free. Or at least, as free as I can be.

The woman who returns my belongings kindly arranges a taxi. My phone is dead, and I can't contact anyone, but I don't have the energy to care. She hands me my few possessions, and I take them with a shaky sigh of relief.

Among them are my sunglasses—one arm missing, the frame cracked—but they feel precious. I slide them onto my face anyway, grateful for anything to shield me from the world, to hide the swollen mess of my eyes. It's a small comfort, but right now, I'll take it.

I step into the midday sun. The light hits me like a wave—blinding, hot, almost suffocating. After hours in fluorescent chill, the warmth on my skin is pure bliss. Real. Alive. I squint and breathe.

The street feels surreal. My sandals slap the pavement, the broken sunglasses perched awkwardly on my face. Construction noise fills the air—machines clanking, voices shouting. I walk the two blocks to meet the taxi, disoriented but determined. This strange, tentative freedom feels fragile, but real.

The driver takes me downtown, to where I'd parked nearly 24 hours earlier. This is a town I've loved and lived in for two decades—a place where I raised my kids, built a life, felt safe. But everything looks unfamiliar now, like a dream where nothing quite fits.

Just yesterday, I strolled these same streets without a care. I remember the cold pint of beer—my usual—grabbed at a local pub before heading next door to eat. That ordinary moment now feels like it belonged to someone else.

The cab drops me a block from my car. As I step onto the sidewalk, a fresh wave of shame rushes in. I scan the street as I lower my head, praying I don't run into anyone I know. I'm not ready for questions—or worse, assumptions.

I reach my car in seconds. There's a parking ticket tucked under the wiper—a mundane reminder of the life I used to live. It feels almost comical. Cruel, even. I barely care.

I slide into the driver's seat and close the door. The quiet hum of the car, the feel of the steering wheel in my hands—it's all shockingly normal. Like I've landed back in a version of my life I no longer recognize. Still, there's something grounding in the familiarity.

For the first time in hours, I'm in control. I can go home. I can see my dog. Just thinking of her—tail wagging, eyes full of love—almost breaks me. I start the car and take a long, shaky breath. It's not over. But I'm going home.

The four-minute drive is a blur—part relief, part panic. I pull up in front of my house and practically run to the front steps, unsure of what I'll find.

Is Mimi stressed? Does she need water? Is she okay?

I open the door. She hops groggily down from her leather chair, stretches, and trots over like it's just another day. No barking. No panic. Just her usual happy greeting.

I check her bowls—both full. Relief washes over me.

She's okay.

I breathe deeply and scan the room. My cats are curled up, their bodies relaxed and warm, sleeping peacefully. Unbothered. Their calm feels like a miracle. It's the first moment of peace I've had in nearly 24 hours.

I charge my phone just enough to make a call. I dial Natasha. The words pour out—broken, frantic, raw. She listens quietly, her voice steady and soothing. Within minutes, she's at my door.

Without a word, she heads to the kitchen and starts cooking with whatever she finds. I can barely eat, but I know I need something. As I force down a few bites, she rubs my arms and legs—gentle, grounding. Her quiet presence is the only thing keeping me tethered.

"It's going to be okay," she says softly. "This must be some horrible mistake."

I want to believe her. But deep down, I know—I don't know anything anymore. I'm here. I'm breathing. That's all I've got.

After she leaves, I crawl into my daughter's bed with the animals. It's the only place that feels safe. Their bodies pressed against mine, the soft hum of their breathing lulls me to sleep. When I wake, it's as if I've been gone for years.

Eventually, I call my employer—my friend and mentor. I can't avoid it any longer. I tell her everything. There's no way to sugarcoat it: I woke up in a hospital, injured, arrested for battery and criminal threat, then jailed. Her shock is palpable, but she listens.

In the days that follow, I barely move. I walk the dog, eat a little, try to watch TV. I am numb—physically, emotionally. I know the facts: I've been charged with violent crimes. My bruised face mirrors my broken spirit. But none of it makes sense.

I hire a criminal defense attorney. He reassures me he'll help. I don't need to attend the first court date—"Just focus on taking care of yourself and your children," he says. I pay him $10,000. Between bail and legal fees, I'm down $20,000 in a matter of hours. But none of it feels real. I would've paid anything not to return to that place.

Still, the unease lingers. The days blur. I drift in limbo—confused, grieving, afraid. Every decision feels too heavy to make.

Then, four days later, it hits me like a freight train: I was drugged.

Up until that point, my mind had been too foggy to process anything clearly. I likely had a concussion—the hospital never ruled it out. My thinking was slow, disjointed. Everything felt scrambled. But something shifts. A crack of clarity opens.

I remember: It was around 3 p.m. I'd stopped for a pint at the bar next to the restaurant where I planned to eat—a ritual I'd done countless times in my life. I'd worked in bars and restaurants for years in my youth. That world felt familiar, easy. I didn't think twice.

I was 50. Capable. Confident. I knew my limits. I was used to alcohol, especially just a beer or two. I'd never blacked out. Not in college. Not ever. I'd never become aggressive. Never lost time.

None of it made sense.

And then a memory flashes—sharp and sudden. A man. Loud, crude, cocky. Sitting with two others. Their energy was off—hostile, almost aggressive. I clocked it, but brushed it off.

About 30 minutes in, I was sipping my beer, editing photos on my phone. I must've sensed something—someone—behind me, because I remember turning to look.

It was him. That man.

He was standing too close. His eyes locked onto mine—not casually, but deliberately. His whole posture was squared toward me, leaning in, staring—like he was studying me. Studying my eyes.

That was my last memory.

I checked my credit card: two beers. A tip. Standard. After that—nothing.

But it was the only memory I needed. With every fiber of my body, I knew: He had drugged me.

He was watching for signs it had taken effect. Studying my pupils. Expecting me to black out; he must have assumed I wouldn't remember.

But I did. Clear as day.

Another detail surfaced—my body reacts slowly to medication. It always has. Maybe he was wondering what was taking so long, watching for signs I'd been affected by whatever I'd unknowingly ingested.

Now it all made sense. The missing hours, the strange behavior, the complete loss of control—it wasn't me. I had been chemically hijacked.

It was the explanation I'd been searching for. I called my attorney, full of hope. I told him everything.

He listened. Said he believed me—but sounded unmoved. My word, my knowing, wasn't enough. The bar hadn't preserved video footage. It would be my word against theirs, with nothing to support what I knew in my bones.

He even cautioned that bringing it up—claiming involuntary intoxication—could backfire. It might make me seem "unaccountable," like I was dodging responsibility.

And just like that, the relief evaporated. My truth—raw, terrifying, clear—would likely never be enough.

CHAPTER 4 | UNFATHOMABLE

I reached out again to my employer—an ER doctor with years of experience at the very hospital where I'd been taken by ambulance. I told her what had come flooding back: the memory, the certainty I'd been drugged. She didn't hesitate. She agreed. The signs were unmistakable—complete amnesia, vomiting, erratic behavior. With my consent, she offered to look into my toxicology screen.

When she called me back, her words hit like a punch: no toxicology screen had been performed. No rape kit. Nothing. The attending physician had diagnosed alcohol intoxication, attributing my deep lacerations and bruising to a fall.

That was the version the arresting officer gave the hospital—and it was accepted without question.

I was stunned. As a clinician, I knew what protocols should have been followed. I was injured, confused, agitated. Why hadn't they tested for drugs?

Why didn't anyone examine my body or follow even the most basic trauma procedures? I had lived by those standards. I knew they'd been ignored.

When I raised concerns with hospital staff, I was met with indifference. They pointed to my elevated blood alcohol level and insisted they'd done nothing wrong.

It was almost impossible to process. These were trained professionals—colleagues in a system I had served for decades. But I hadn't been treated as a patient in crisis. I was treated as a problem. Labeled the "assailant," and handled accordingly.

What I didn't know at the time was that I'd been heavily sedated during much of my stay. A CT scan was done, likely due to head trauma. Three deep facial wounds were sutured. Then I was discharged—in handcuffs.

Later, I reviewed the body cam footage. I watched myself—confused, bloodied—repeating that I had been assaulted. No one listened. My words were dismissed.

It felt like a second violation. I wasn't seen as someone in need of care—I was written off as just another intoxicated woman who'd gone too far. I filed a formal complaint with the hospital, hoping for accountability. Nothing came of it.

Reading my medical records was gut-wrenching. I was described as "confused," repeatedly asking the same questions. Yet no one questioned the origin of my injuries. No tests. No follow-up. Just a narrative accepted without scrutiny.

I consulted civil attorneys about the hospital's negligence and the police's superficial investigation. The answer was always the same: I didn't have a case.

There is no law requiring drug testing or the administration of a rape kit. The hospital staff said they had no reason to suspect I'd been victimized—even though I was badly injured, disoriented, and required sedation. Because of that, they concluded there had been no wrongdoing.

For weeks, the only story I had was the one the police gave me: that I'd assaulted someone and then fallen, causing my injuries. I had no memory to dispute it.

Then my attorneys said something that changed everything—I was the one who called 911. No one else had contacted the police. The story that I'd attacked someone only emerged after officers arrived. They had been responding to my call for help.

Eventually, two witnesses came forward. One had seen a man throw me out of the bar—already bloodied, before I hit the ground. Another remembered me vomiting, then being immediately assaulted by several individuals. Neither described my behavior as aggressive.

There had been no "citizen's arrest," despite that being documented in my medical record. I wasn't restrained for safety. I was beaten—badly—by multiple male patrons at a place of business. And I had been the one who called for help.

I listened to the 911 call. My voice was clearer than I expected. I said I'd been attacked. The fear was unmistakable. I had believed someone would listen.

But the officers accepted the version offered by bystanders—regulars at the bar, some of whom I now suspect were involved. Despite my significant injuries—clearly inconsistent with a simple fall—and despite the 911 call and body cam footage where I repeatedly said I had been attacked, I was the only one arrested. No surveillance footage was preserved. The bar was never treated as a crime scene. The investigation—if you could call it that—was cursory at best.

Later, I learned the person identified as the "victim" was an employee at the bar where I'd been attacked. The others? Regular patrons with ties to the establishment—or to law enforcement.

My call for help placed me at the mercy of a system more invested in protecting itself than seeking the truth.

It was devastating. Had I stayed silent, none of this would have happened. Instead of being protected, I was punished.

Despite the evidence—witnesses, medical records, the 911 call, body cam footage—the DA pursued charges against me.

"It's clear you were assaulted," my attorney said. "There's no way this will go to trial."

He was wrong.

In court, I sat labeled as the defendant while the DA painted me as unstable and aggressive—never once acknowledging that I had been the one to call 911. That I had been seriously injured.

The employee who accused me of starting the altercation was friends with the man identified as the primary assailant—the one who split my face in several places. The man who, I later learned, had punched me repeatedly while I was on the floor.

I had to see him again and again in court, always seated beside the person referred to as *"the victim."* That title was never given to me. Not once was I acknowledged as someone who had been harmed. No one ever asked me what I had experienced. My trauma wasn't even named.

That silence—the refusal to see me—was its own kind of violence.

More than a year after the event, a chilling thought took hold: I may have been drugged with the intent to be trafficked.

The day after I was released, I received a text from a man I didn't recognize. He claimed we'd spoken outside the bar for over an hour and said he'd left me around 5:30 p.m. I had no memory of him—none.

I asked him to meet, hoping that something would come back to me. My face was still stitched and bruised when we sat down. I told him I'd been arrested and had no memory of our interaction.

His reaction was strange—eerily detached. He didn't ask a single question. No concern, no curiosity, no acknowledgment of what I'd just shared. Instead, he launched into casual talk about yoga, California, himself. The conversation floated on the surface, as if nothing significant had happened.

It was an oddly flat response. If someone told me they'd been badly beaten and had no memory of an hour-long conversation we'd had, I would've been shocked—concerned, at the very least.

I wanted to believe him. For a while, I did.

I reviewed the police report. The first documented incident was at 8:33 p.m.—nearly three hours after he said he'd left me. That gap changed everything. Where had I been for all those hours?

I remembered that when I asked him to meet, I had experienced a visceral wave of repulsion. I didn't remember him consciously, but my body must have known something.

He'd been messaging me every few months from different cities—vague check-ins I hadn't thought much of—until then. Was he keeping tabs? Gauging what I remembered?

I sent him a message, saying I was starting to remember more and asked if we could talk. He didn't respond. I followed up. He had always responded quickly to me in the past; this was out of character. Read receipts confirmed he saw my text messages.

Then he blocked me.

His silence said everything.

I shared all of this with my attorneys. It didn't matter. No hard proof. No case.

I later learned the area where I was drugged had a well-documented history of crime. The bar was one of the most heavily policed in the city. Not long after my incident, another patron was violently assaulted by employees—caught on camera. Eventually, the city shut the place down.

It changed nothing for me.

The DA pressed forward. I was a single mother, a career nurse with a spotless record—and still, I was treated as the threat.

My attorneys advised me not to pursue criminal or civil action until the charges were resolved. Regretfully, I listened. As the case dragged on, the statute of limitations came and went. I never even filed a police report.

Eighteen months later, after weeks in trial, the case ended in a mistrial. Still, the DA wouldn't drop it. More delays. It could be another year. In the end, truth seemed irrelevant.

That's when I chose to speak out. I created a TikTok account and shared my story. It was terrifying—but necessary. If I stayed silent, I felt I would die. I needed to start expressing what had happened to me. I needed to get it out of my body.

My attorneys withdrew representation when they found out. They sent me an email that alluded to some fine print in our contract that released them from their legal obligation. After paying them over $25,000, I was left completely alone.

That's when I understood: there would be no justice.

I had been drugged, possibly trafficked, assaulted, arrested, and publicly shamed—and no one in the *system* seemed to care.

Then the Board of Registered Nursing came after my license. After 23 years of a spotless record, I was suddenly under investigation.

Nursing had been my identity. My livelihood. My security. And now, I was facing yet another battle I never saw coming.

Consulting an expert attorney revealed that the only way to share my story with the board was an administrative hearing—and that I would be responsible for not only my own legal fees but theirs too, likely $30–60K. An impossible burden with resources I simply didn't have."

The alternative? A five-year drug and alcohol rehab program. I'd have to shut down my skincare business, resign from my director-role at a clinic, undergo constant assessments and monitoring, and live under the assumption that I was unwell—until the board *deemed* otherwise.

It felt surreal. I had no record of substance use, no workplace issues, no prior record. And still, I was swiftly and decisively cast as the problem.

It didn't matter that I knew exactly what had happened, where it had occurred, and who was responsible for harming me—or that the businesses where I'd been targeted, had a documented pattern of violent crime.

I submitted a written statement. Friends and colleagues stood beside me with letters of support. Still, there was no acknowledgment—no confirmation that any of it was ever received, let alone read.

With no resources left, and a deep knowing that I couldn't agree to their terms, I surrendered my nursing license—and with it, I let go of my livelihood, my sense of safety, and a role that had been a core part of my identity for over twenty years.

CHAPTER 5 | A NEW FIGHT

Letting go of my professional license after more than two decades cut deep—but it also set me free. Nursing had been at the center of who I was. But staying would have meant accepting a story that erased the truth. Walking away felt like the only choice—a declaration: I wouldn't betray myself. I would build something new, something real, wholly my own. I stopped waiting to be heard, waiting for justice. Instead, I became the one who listened.

The trauma felt vast, archetypal. The ultimate gaslighting—being harmed and then blamed—echoed patterns I had carried my whole life: bearing what wasn't mine, living within constructs I never accepted, wearing masks that kept me separate. The assault didn't break me. It burned away what I had outgrown: illusions, routines that felt safe but stifling, narratives I no longer recognized as mine. It left me raw, awake, ready.

Weeks before it happened, I had stood on a hillside, overlooking my home, whispering a prayer—to God, to the trees, to anyone listening. I asked for a life more aligned with my heart, my soul, my truest self. I didn't know then that those words planted a spark, a small flame that would ignite a shedding so complete it felt like demolition. From those ashes, I began to build again—stronger, truer, entirely on my own foundation.

I started trusting myself again—my body, my beliefs, my intuition. I reconnected with the quiet inner knowing that speaks beyond words. Breathwork became my lifeline: at first, just a way to soothe my nervous system, then a portal back to myself.

I added other practices—movement in nature, journaling, sitting in silence. Simple rituals that reminded me who I was, that beauty and joy existed even in pain.

Healing didn't come from grand gestures. It came from being okay with myself, noticing what was present, and meeting it with attention and compassion. Some people faded from my life. That hurt. But deeper, more authentic connections emerged—people who could meet me where I truly was.

Sharing my story became an act of healing, resistance, and radical self-love. Slowly, I realized: I was no longer just surviving.

Breath, movement, expression, connection—they became my anchors in the storm. They brought me back to my center, to myself. And from this place, I rediscovered peace. I found clarity, and something else long forgotten: freedom. Not the kind granted by a system, but the kind that can only be created from within.

PART TWO | BRIDGE AND ANCHOR: BREATHING WITH ATTENTION AND INTENTION

"Feelings come and go like clouds in a windy sky. Conscious breathing is my anchor."

—Thich Nhat Hanh."

After the assault, my body wouldn't settle. Sleep was fitful, appetite inconsistent, and my thoughts scattered. Panic and racing heartbeats became regular, and the coping tools I'd relied on—therapy, walks, time with friends—weren't enough to restore calm. I realized I didn't need more thinking. I needed a new baseline.

Breathwork became that baseline. Simple, intentional breathing offered steadiness when everything else felt chaotic. At first, it was about survival—just a few minutes at a time. Gradually, it became a way to return to myself and access safety in my body again.

The breath asks for nothing and gives everything. No rules, no labels, no explanation—just your attention, and it will meet you wherever you are.

This section isn't a medical guide. It's a companion for reclaiming your inner calm, for steadying your nervous system, and for finding your own rhythm in the midst of life's storms. It's rooted in my experience as a nurse, my training in trauma-informed breathwork, and, most importantly, my lived journey.

Along the way, I also came to understand the science behind why these practices work—the nervous system, heart-brain connection, and the physiology of breath. Knowing the "why" doesn't replace the practice, but it offers clarity, reassurance, and a framework to deepen your experience.

Let it meet you where you are.

CHAPTER 6 | THE WISDOM OF REGULATION

When your nervous system is dysregulated, it's easy to think something is wrong with you—that you're too anxious, too numb, too "off." The truth is, your body isn't broken. It's responding. And one of the fastest ways to help it reset is through your breath.

Your body is designed to keep you safe. At the heart of this system is your nervous system—a vast network constantly scanning both your inner and outer world for safety or threat.

This process, called neuroception (coined by Dr. Stephen Porges in his Polyvagal Theory), happens automatically, without conscious thought.

Safety: Your nervous system allows you to be calm, connected, and present.

Perceived danger: Your body prepares to fight, flee, or shut down.

Dysregulation: When the system gets stuck in survival mode, it can't easily return to baseline.

Your body's reactions—your overwhelm, irritability, or emotional flatness—are survival mechanisms, not failures.

BREATH: YOUR BUILT-IN MEDICINE

Breath is always with you, from your first cry to your final exhale. Simple, ordinary, but incredibly powerful. Breathwork is the practice of turning inward with intention, using your breath to regulate your nervous system, release emotion, and strengthen self-trust.

According to Giten Tonkov, founder of Biodynamic Breathwork and the Trauma Release System, the breath offers a doorway—an entryway not just to calm, but to profound inner transformation.

ANCIENT WISDOM; MODERN SCIENCE

Breathwork is nothing new. Yogic pranayama, Taoist breathing, and Indigenous traditions have long honored the breath as sacred medicine—a bridge between body, mind, and spirit.

Modern research now confirms these benefits. As James Nestor highlights in *Breath*, slow, conscious breathing activates the parasympathetic nervous system, our rest-and-restore mode. It lowers heart rate, reduces cortisol, supports digestion, and tells the body: *You're safe now.*

Shallow, rapid breathing, by contrast, keeps the body in fight-or-flight, locked in stress. Conscious breath interrupts that loop, sending a new message: *I am safe.*

THE VAGUS NERVE: YOUR INNER REGULATOR

The vagus nerve, the longest cranial nerve, runs from your brainstem through your heart, lungs, and gut. It's a key player in regulating breath, digestion, inflammation, and emotion.

According to Dr. Porges' Polyvagal Theory, the nervous system moves through three states:

Ventral vagal (safe + social): grounded, calm, connected

Sympathetic (fight or flight): anxious, activated

Dorsal vagal (shutdown): numb, frozen, disconnected

Flexibility—the ability to move between states and return to baseline—is what matters most. Breathwork supports that flexibility.

THE BODY SPEAKS TO THE BRAIN

About 80% of vagal signals move from body to brain, meaning your body constantly informs your mind.

Shallow breath → brain interprets danger → stress response

Slow, deep breath → brain receives safety cues → calm and clarity

As Dr. Bessel van der Kolk explains in *The Body Keeps the Score,* trauma is stored in the body. Breath is one of the gentlest ways to create safety and invite healing.

BREATH, INFLAMMATION AND IMMUNITY

Low vagal tone is linked to chronic inflammation, which affects immunity, cardiovascular health, and mood. Breath practices—especially slow, long exhalations—activate the vagus nerve, reducing inflammation and supporting resilience.

Other vagus-friendly tools include:

- Cold exposure (splashes of water, cold showers)
- Humming, chanting, or singing
- Deep belly laughter or gargling

BREATH, CO2, AND OXYGEN

Better breathing isn't about "more oxygen," but about using it efficiently. The Bohr Effect explains that carbon dioxide (CO_2) helps release oxygen into your tissues. Chronic over-breathing expels too much CO_2, reducing oxygen delivery. Practices like box breathing or gentle breath holds improve CO_2 tolerance and restore balance (Patrick McKeown, *The Oxygen Advantage*).

STRESS AND THE BRAIN

Chronic stress reshapes the brain:

Shrinks the hippocampus (memory)

Weakens the prefrontal cortex (decision-making, regulation)

Hyper-activates the amygdala (constant threat scanning)

The good news? The brain is plastic. Intentional breath soothes the amygdala, strengthens the prefrontal cortex, and recalibrates your baseline. Over time, you feel calmer, more responsive, and less reactive.

KEY TAKEAWAYS: CHAPTER 6

Dysregulation isn't failure; it's survival. Your nervous system is protecting you.

Breath is a built-in medicine for regulation, emotional balance, and resilience.

Ancient practices and modern science converge: slow, conscious breath calms, heals, and restores.

The vagus nerve is your reset button. Supporting it creates safety and connection.

Your body communicates with your brain. Slow breath rewires thought, emotion, and state.

A few minutes of conscious breathing daily can shift your baseline, calm your body, and reconnect you to yourself.

BREATHING PRACTICE: SLOW RHYTHMIC BREATHING

Theme: Nervous system regulation, emotional balance, grounded presence

Duration: 5–10 minutes (or longer if desired)

When to Use:

- During stress, anxiety, or overwhelm
- Before important conversations or decisions
- Daily, to build resilience and restore balance

PRACTICE INSTRUCTIONS:

1. Set the Space: Sit or lie comfortably. Let your body feel supported.
2. Set an Intention: e.g., "I choose calm," or "My breath is safe."
3. Begin the Breath: Inhale through the nose for 4–5 counts, letting the breath reach your belly. Exhale through the nose for 6 or longer—slightly longer than the inhale.
4. Stay With It: Maintain the rhythm. Return to the count if your mind wanders. Notice softening in your body.
5. Adjust as Needed: Skip counting if it feels rigid; focus on elongating the exhale.
6. Close the Practice: Release the count, breathe naturally, place hands on heart or belly, and notice the shift.

INQUIRY PROMPT:

How did your body or emotions respond?

What signals did your nervous system give before and after?

What might become possible when calm is your baseline?

CHAPTER 7 | THE RITUAL OF RETURN

We often think of healing as dramatic—a breakthrough, a rock-bottom moment, a bold leap forward. But real transformation usually happens quietly, in the small, steady choices we make every day. It happens in those ordinary moments when we turn inward, soften, and simply return to ourselves.

This chapter is about those moments.

Here, breathwork becomes less about learning a new skill and more about remembering an innate one. It's a way to unbrace your body, untangle emotional knots you may not even know you're carrying, and reconnect with the gentle wisdom of your breath—especially when life feels heavy, relentless, or out of control.

This isn't about doing more. It's about doing differently.

Breathing differently.

Breathwork meets you exactly where you are—in your overwhelm, grief, insomnia—and begins to shift something quietly from within. It asks only that you show up, one breath at a time.

In this chapter, you'll see how breath supports emotional release, deep rest, and resilience without requiring perfect conditions or hours of time. You'll also learn how to integrate it into everyday life, making it a quiet but powerful ally in healing.

BREATH AS A GATEWAY TO FEELING

In my own healing journey, breathwork didn't just calm me—it helped me *feel*. Each inhale and exhale opened a door into my emotional body, revealing truths buried beneath survival.

Think about what happens after stress: your stomach knots, your jaw clenches. These aren't random—they're protective responses. When tension lingers, it hardens into emotional armor.

Breathwork helps release what the body holds. Unprocessed emotions—especially trauma, grief, or chronic stress—often show up as pain, tension, or numbness. Somatic research confirms what we intuitively know: the body remembers, and the breath can help reset it when we get stuck in dysregulation.

The vagus nerve, the messenger between body and brain, plays a central role in processing stress and emotion. Breathwork shifts the nervous system out of defense and back into connection. It doesn't ask you to name what's rising—it simply invites you to feel it.

Warmth in the chest, tingling in the limbs, waves of emotion without a clear story—these are signs your nervous system is unwinding.

Different practices meet us in different ways. Structured methods like Holotropic or Conscious Connected Breathing can create deep release, while gentler practices like Box Breathing or Coherent Breathing support grounding and regulation.

As Dr. Stephen Porges notes, these methods support heart rate variability (HRV)—a key measure of resilience.

Over time, breath softens the protective layers that once kept you safe but also kept you distant from yourself.

THE BREATH AS A BRIDGE TO SLEEP

For years, I struggled to sleep. Even when exhausted, my mind would spin—replaying the day, planning the next, bracing for the worst.

Your breath is one of the most powerful ways to signal safety. Slow, intentional breathing tells your body: *You're safe now. You can rest.* It lowers cortisol, supports melatonin, calms heart rate, and relaxes muscle tension. In sleep science, this is called "downshifting arousal"—and breath supports it beautifully.

The beauty is that we can start simply. Even just lengthening the exhale, stimulates the vagus nerve and signals safety. Over time, your breath becomes a cue: *it's safe to let go, it is time to sleep.*

Research on Coherent Breathing (around 5–6 breaths per minute) shows improved HRV, better sleep quality, and reduced insomnia symptoms (Lehrer et al., 2020).

A simple ritual I love: dim the lights, put away screens, and take a few minutes of intentional breathing before bed. Not to be productive—but to give your body permission to rest. This isn't just more sleep—it's better sleep. The kind that restores, integrates, and heals.

INTEGRATING BREATHWORK INTO EVERYDAY LIFE

Life doesn't pause so we can catch our breath. But breath lets us root within it—finding stillness in motion.

You don't need an hour, a special room, or an altar. You can begin exactly where you are. One client—a full-time professional and mother—called breathwork her sanctuary. Not in long rituals, but in micro-moments: before school drop-off, between meetings, while cooking dinner. She didn't create more time—she reclaimed it.

Breathwork in real life might look like:

- A few grounding breaths on your morning commute
- Syncing breath while folding laundry
- Pausing to breathe fully at a red light
- One or two deep belly breaths before answering an email

Each breath interrupts the default stress pattern. It creates a choice instead of a reaction. As Deb Dana writes in *Anchored*, these small practices support regulation and build trust in your nervous system.

The more you return to your breath, the more resilient you become. Your nervous system learns to move between activation and calm with greater ease. That's neuroplasticity in real time.

A PRACTICE OF PATIENCE AND PRESENCE

Healing isn't linear. Emotional release doesn't happen all at once. Breathwork unfolds in layers—moment by moment.

Your capacity grows over time. Your nervous system strengthens. You begin to meet yourself with compassion.

This is not a performance. There's no "right" way to breathe. You're not chasing a breakthrough—you're building a relationship. Set your pace. Set your boundaries. Be kind to yourself.

Each breath is an act of kindness—a way to meet discomfort with curiosity, not fear. As Dr. Kristin Neff reminds us in *Self-Compassion*, gentleness is not weakness—it's power.

Whether you're seeking emotional healing, better sleep, or a way to stay grounded, breathwork offers the same message again and again:

You are safe.
You are here.

You can return to yourself.

KEY TAKEAWAYS: CHAPTER 7

Breathwork supports emotional healing by releasing stuck emotions and reconnecting you with your body.

Conscious breathing downshifts the system into rest, improving sleep and hormonal balance.

Integrating micro-practices woven into daily life build regulation and resilience.

Breathwork builds resilience and strengthens the nervous system's capacity to recover and adapt.

Breath is your most accessible healing tool—always available, always free.

Healing is slow alchemy. Let your breath guide you gently, steadily, faithfully.

BREATHING PRACTICE: OCEAN BREATH (UJJAYI)

Theme: Deep rest, nervous system reset, inner quiet
Duration: 8–12 minutes (or longer if desired)

When to Use:

- As a wind-down before bed
- After emotionally or physically demanding moments
- Anytime you feel overstimulated

Practice:

1. Set the Space: Dim lights, sit or recline comfortably. Allow your body to feel supported.
2. Set an Intention: e.g., "I welcome rest," or "I return to calm."
3. Find the Rhythm: Keep the breath slow, steady, and even. Let the ocean sound anchor your attention.

4. Stay With It: Follow the sensation and sound of your breath. If thoughts arise, gently return to the rhythm. Allow your breath to soften your body.
5. Adjust as Needed: If constriction feels challenging, simply breathe slowly through the nose. No need to force the sound.
6. Close the Practice: Release the constriction, return to natural breathing, rest, and notice how your body feels. Let your breath integrate.

INQUIRY PROMPT:

- What shifted in my body or mind during this practice?
- How do I feel now compared to before?
- How might I allow rest to become a regular part of my healing?

CHAPTER 8 | THE ALCHEMY OF EMOTION

Breathing is life's most constant rhythm—happening over 20,000 times a day, often without conscious thought. Beneath this steady pulse lies something profound: an untapped source of emotional clarity, insight, and inner knowing.

Breathwork doesn't just support rest and regulation—it opens the door to deeper truths. It helps us meet emotions we've avoided, rediscover parts of ourselves we may have abandoned, and gently reclaim them. The breath becomes both a healing balm and a mirror, revealing who we are beneath the noise of daily life.

In this chapter, we'll explore the living anatomy of breath, how stress and trauma shape breathing patterns, and how intentional breathwork supports emotional regulation, embodiment, and healing.

We'll come to see the breath as a subtle language of emotion—a bridge between inner experience and authentic expression. We'll also touch on how personal breath awareness can ripple outward, affecting collective energy.

THE LIVING ANATOMY OF BREATH: A WHOLE BODY EXPERIENCE

Breath is more than air moving in and out of the lungs—it's a full-body experience, involving muscles, bones, fascia, and nerves working in harmony. Somatic therapies call this embodied breath, where physiological movement meets emotional and energetic flow.

- Diaphragm: This dome-shaped muscle at the base of the ribcage contracts on inhalation and relaxes on exhalation. It supports posture, massages internal organs, aids lymphatic flow, and activates the vagus nerve, signaling safety to the nervous system.
- Lungs: Millions of alveoli allow oxygen into the blood and carbon dioxide out. Breath fuels both body and emotional regulation.
- Rib Cage and Intercostals: Protect the lungs and assist chest expansion. Stress often shifts us to shallow, upper-chest breathing—a common trauma response.
- Pelvic Floor: Works with the diaphragm, relaxing on the inhale and lifting on the exhale. Chronic tension here can reflect emotional constriction.
- Psoas: A deep core muscle often linked to fear and stress. Softening it through breath supports grounding and emotional release. Fascia and muscle memory hold emotional imprints (Schleip, 2020).
- Fascia: This connective web transmits breath's movement throughout the body. Mindful breathing restores its flexibility and flow.
- Circulation and Detox: The diaphragm supports circulation and lymphatic flow, aiding the body's natural healing processes.

HOW STRESS AND TRAUMA SHAPE BREATH

Stress literally narrows the breath. Muscles tighten, the diaphragm constricts, and breathing becomes shallow or frozen. These patterns often become habitual when trauma remains unresolved.

Common stress patterns include:

Shallow chest breathing: Signals hypervigilance

Breath holding: A freeze response linked to fear or grief

Paradoxical breathing: Disconnection between belly and chest

These are not flaws—they are adaptations. Breathwork invites the body out of defense and back into flow.

Emotional Signatures in Breath:

Anxiety: Short, rapid breaths

Grief: Held breath or sighs

Calm: Softened, slower rhythm

Try this check-in: Place one hand on your belly, one on your chest. Where does the breath move most easily? Can you feel your ribs, back, and pelvis responding? Imagine your breath as a gentle wave moving through your whole body. Learning to listen—*interoception*—is foundational to emotional healing (Mehling et al., 2012).

BREATH AS EMOTIONAL LANGUAGE

Each emotion has its own signature. Breathwork creates space for them to arise, move through, and complete.

We don't have to analyze every sensation—we simply stay present long enough to let them move. Over time, breath builds the capacity to feel without being consumed, to soften and meet what is present, rather than brace.

Some practices that support emotional well-being:

- Breath Awareness: Soft attention to your natural rhythm
- Diaphragmatic Breathing: Deepens regulation via the vagus nerve
- Box Breathing: Structured rhythm to calm anxiety
- Coherent Breathing: Balances HRV and steadies the nervous system
- Somatic Breathwork: For deeper emotional release

Physical responses—tingling, tears, warmth—are normal. Go slowly. Be kind. Trauma survivors may benefit from a trauma-informed facilitator (Levine, *In an Unspoken Voice*).

THE BREATH AS A MIRROR

Breath reveals what's hidden: tension in the jaw, numbness in the belly, longing in the chest. These are entry points, not obstacles. Staying with the breath allows these truths to soften.

Healing doesn't mean eliminating pain—it means learning how to meet it. The breath shows us how.

Breathing through transition:

Grief: Slow exhales hold space for sorrow

Anxiety: Box breathing provides stability

Heartbreak: Coherent breath nurtures compassion

FROM PERSONAL PRACTICE TO COLLECTIVE BREATH

When we breathe with presence, we affect more than ourselves. Group breathwork demonstrates this: shared rhythms, strangers exhaling in unison. Safety expands.

You don't need to be a teacher. Your regulated breath becomes an invitation to those around you—a ripple effect of calm and connection (Porges, *The Pocket Guide to Polyvagal Theory*).

KEY TAKEAWAYS: CHAPTER 8

Breath is a full-body experience, shaped by emotion, fascia, and nervous system state

Stress patterns alter breath, but they can be unwound

Breathwork bridges inner awareness and healing

Each breath carries an emotional signature that reveals and reshapes patterns

Breath anchors us through transitions and moments of change

Collective breath creates a ripple effect of regulation and connection

BREATHING PRACTICE: CONSCIOUS CONNECTED BREATH

Theme: Energizing the body, emotional release, and shifting stuck patterns
Duration: 10–15 minutes (adjust as needed)

When to Use:

- Feeling emotionally stuck or overwhelmed
- Needing a reset or energetic shift
- Morning or midday re-centering

PRACTICE INSTRUCTIONS:

1. Set the Space: Lie down in a safe, quiet place. Let your body feel supported.

2. Set an Intention: e.g., "I welcome release" or "I trust my breath."

3. Begin the Breath: Inhale through the mouth into the belly and chest.

4. Exhale softly without pausing. Keep the breath circular and connected.

5. Stay With It: Let the breath carry you. If emotion arises, stay present.

6. Soften your jaw and shoulders and anywhere else you notice tension.

7. Adjust if Needed: Slow down or switch to nose breathing at any time.

8. Close the Practice: After 8–10 minutes, return to natural breathing.

9. Rest quietly. Place your hands on heart and belly. Feel the shift.

INQUIRY PROMPT: BREATH AS BREAKTHROUGH

>   What moved or softened?
>
>   What emotions or memories surfaced?
>
>   What resistance did I notice, and what helped me stay with it?
>
>   Let your journaling be free and unfiltered. Breathe into what you find.

PART THREE | THE LIFELINES: THREADS OF RETURN AND REMEMBRANCE

"Take your broken heart, make it into art."

— Carrie Fisher

WHAT ARE THE LIFELINES?

Breathwork became my anchor, but it wasn't the whole story. What carried me forward was a constellation of simple, steady practices—rituals I returned to again and again to feel safe, grounded, and whole. These practices became my Lifelines: heart-centered tools that helped me reclaim myself, piece by piece.

The Lifelines aren't rules or checklists. They aren't a formula for "success." They are living, intuitive practices—anchors that bring you back to your body, your breath, and your strength. Each speaks to a different part of healing: from nervous system regulation to emotional expression, from embodied presence to spiritual reconnection. Together, they form a flexible framework for steady restoration.

WHY THEY MATTER

If breathwork is the roadmap back to yourself, the Lifelines are the lanterns lighting the path. They are accessible touchstones you can reach for when you feel unmoored, overwhelmed, or lost. They help you return to your own rhythm, honoring your story, your nervous system, and your pace. Healing doesn't come from force—it comes from repeated, small acts of care.

Start where you are. You don't need to practice them all at once. You don't need to master anything. Let each one meet you here. Healing unfolds at the pace of trust, and the Lifelines are here to guide you.

THE LIFELINES

These practices became my steady companions through the storm:

- Radical Self-Love – You are Enough.
- Feel All Your Feelings – They are Meant to be Felt.
- Bend – Move your Body and Let it Move You.

- Breathe – Come Back to your Center.
- Sound – Listen deeply. Express Freely.
- Circle – Be Held. Hold Others.
- Express – Let your Truth be Seen.
- Heart & Hands – Service, Gratitude, and Trust.
- Body Temple – Care for the Vessel that Carries you.

In the pages that follow, I'll share the tools, reflections, and practices that helped me rebuild from the inside out. My hope is that you find something here to steady you—something that reminds you:

You are not broken.

You are reclaiming.

You are becoming.

CHAPTER 9 | RADICAL SELF-LOVE–YOU ARE ENOUGH

Radical self-love is the deep, unshakable belief in your inherent worth—regardless of past mistakes, flaws, or imperfections. It's the practice of offering yourself the same compassion you'd extend to someone you love. It's embracing who you are right now, without waiting to become someone "better."

Self-love isn't a luxury—it's essential. Without it, true healing remains out of reach. Radical self-love disrupts the cycle of shame, self-criticism, and guilt. It's an act of resistance in a world that tells us we must earn our worth. It becomes the foundation for making peace with ourselves—and that is where I began.

When you accept yourself fully, you stop chasing validation. You free yourself from the exhausting need for approval. You begin to trust that your value is intrinsic—not conditional or externally assigned.

HOW THIS LIFELINE SUPPORTS HEALING

- Clears shame and guilt that block progress
- Fosters compassion for your struggles, making healing more accessible

- Invites peace and acceptance, allowing you to move forward with confidence

HOW I LEARNED TO LOVE MYSELF

At first, self-love felt abstract. I understood it intellectually, but I didn't know how to live it. It wasn't about bubble baths or pedicures—though those can help. It was deeper.

Self-love became how I showed up for myself when no one else did. How I treated myself in silence. How I spoke to myself in the dark. How I held onto my worth when everything else felt like it was falling apart.

In the early days of healing, isolation was sharp. The people I once leaned on were absent—or unable to meet me in my pain. No one was coming to save me. The institutions, friendships, and systems I had trusted couldn't fix what had been broken. That didn't make it easier—but it made it clear: if I was going to move forward, it had to come from within.

After being victimized and then criminalized, I experienced a disorienting abandonment. Many accepted the surface narrative without question. Assumptions spread fast. For someone who had spent her life trying to be understood, it was crushing. I felt judged, humiliated, and unseen.

But within that pain, something powerful emerged: I began to lean into my own knowing. The only opinion that truly mattered was my own. I had to stop managing how others saw me. That shift wasn't easy—but it was liberating.

As Mel Robbins writes in *The Let Them Theory*:
"The truth is, other people's opinions of you are none of your business. Your business is creating the life you want to live."

Letting go of the need to control how others perceived me freed up immense energy—energy I could now direct toward healing, growth, and authentic connection. That was the beginning of radical self-love: not just when it was easy, but especially when it wasn't.

HEALING BEGINS WITH HOW YOU SPEAK TO YOURSELF

The first step was noticing—and gently challenging—my inner voice. It didn't change overnight, but I began catching it.

When I thought, *I'm so alone. This is too hard. Nobody cares,* I paused. Not to deny the pain, but to make room for something more:

> *What if this is hard, but I don't have to go through it unkindly?*
>
> *What if I'm not as alone as I fear?*
>
> *What if I care—and that's enough right now?*

I started speaking to myself the way I would to a hurting friend. I reminded myself I didn't need to earn love through perfection or suffering. I had always carried strength—even humor in darkness—but I began allowing myself softness beneath that strength.

FROM SELF KINDNESS TO INTENTIONAL THOUGHT

Over time, this inner kindness evolved into intentional thought. It became about choosing which thoughts I followed.

Fear often crept in: *What if this goes wrong? I don't know what's coming.*
Instead of spiraling, I paused. *Yes, this is scary. Yes, I don't have all the answers. And still—I choose to trust.*

I began to trust the unfolding. To welcome the mystery. Even for a breath or two, I asked: *What would it feel like to believe life is conspiring for me?*

Where attention goes, energy follows. That quiet shift—from fear to trust, from contraction to openness—has changed everything. This is self-love in action: not just the comforting kind, but the courageous kind that chooses trust, redirects energy, and reframes fear—not to bypass reality, but to reclaim agency.

Breathwork became the anchor for this radical self-love. It gave me the calm and presence I needed to hold these truths.

SELF LOVE IS AN "ACTION WORD"

Radical self-love didn't begin as a feeling—but as a practice. A daily commitment to honoring my worth.

I noticed when I minimized my needs or hesitated to speak up. In those moments, I reminded myself: *You're allowed to take up space. Your voice matters. Your needs are valid.*

One ritual that helped anchor this practice was writing affirmations with my morning coffee. Meeting myself exactly where I was in that moment, I could respond with pen and paper to any feelings of anxiety or fear or sadness..

> *I am enough as I am right now.*
>
> *I trust myself and honor my intuition.*
>
> *I choose where I place my attention.*

Simple, but healing.

This daily check-in helped me meet myself with compassion. Whether overwhelmed by a to-do list or financial stress, I responded with the words I most needed to hear—just as I would for a close friend or child.

Self-love didn't mean putting myself above others. It meant letting my needs matter, too. Releasing the belief that I had to earn love through performance was a profound shift. In that space, I found self-forgiveness. My value isn't in what I produce—it lives in who I am.

BOUNDARIES–A LOVING ACT

One of the clearest expressions of self-love is setting boundaries.

I had always sensed my limits—but learning to honor them consistently, without guilt, changed everything. Boundaries aren't walls. They're guidelines that protect energy and well-being. They don't require drama—just clarity, honesty, and compassion.

At the heart of this is presence: I get to choose where I place my attention. I don't have to absorb every emotion around me. I don't have to say yes to everything. Each boundary I uphold affirms my worth. Protecting my peace isn't selfish—it's sacred.

Through this practice, I've rebuilt my relationship with myself—not just in words, but in how I see myself. I now honor my needs, feelings, and desires—without shame or apology. This is healing: a steady return to myself. In becoming my own ally, I've come home.

THE SCIENCE OF SELF-LOVE

Radical self-love may feel spiritual, but it's also rooted in science. Neuroscience and psychology show that how we relate to ourselves shapes emotional and physical well-being.

Dr. Kristin Neff, a pioneer in self-compassion, found that people who practice it experience less anxiety, depression, and shame—and more resilience. As she writes:
"Self-compassion provides an island of calm, a refuge from the stormy seas of endless positive and negative self-judgment."

Speaking to ourselves with kindness activates the brain's self-soothing system: lowering cortisol and increasing oxytocin, the hormone linked to safety and connection. Positive self-talk also impacts neuroplasticity. As Dr. Rick Hanson writes:
"Neurons that fire together wire together."

Practicing self-love—especially in moments of stress—teaches the brain it's safe to be kind to yourself. Boundaries work biologically, too. They prevent overwhelm, reduce reactivity, and help the nervous system maintain a healthy window of tolerance. Honoring your limits reinforces internal safety.

Self-love is not indulgence—it is regulatory, grounding, and restorative.

REAL LIFE EXAMPLES OF SELF-LOVE

- A woman softens her inner dialogue around body image, writes affirmations like *I love my body for all it does for me*, and practices gratitude after movement. Slowly, her relationship shifts from criticism to respect.

- A man, long conditioned to "always do," starts listening to his body's cues—tight jaw, clenched stomach, mental fatigue. He pauses, reminds himself, *I'm doing the best I can*, and chooses rest without guilt. Each moment becomes an act of permission.

- A woman who habitually says yes to avoid discomfort begins practicing small, clear boundaries. *I don't need to justify my no*, becomes her quiet mantra. She breathes through the discomfort and builds a new sense of safety in her truth.

PRACTICE: MIRROR OF COMPASSION

Look into your own eyes and say:
I love you. You are enough, just as you are.

Repeat several times. Let the words settle. Notice any resistance. Observe without judgment.

If negative thoughts arise, gently respond:
I forgive you. You are worthy of love and grace.

This simple practice reprograms your inner dialogue and deepens your relationship with yourself over time.

CHAPTER 10 | FEEL ALL YOUR FEELINGS—THEY ARE MEANT TO BE FELT

To feel all your feelings means allowing yourself to experience your emotions fully—without judgment, suppression, or avoidance. It's about welcoming the full spectrum of human emotion, from the ones we label "good" to those we resist, with openness and compassion.

Emotions are energy in motion. When we suppress or ignore them, they don't vanish—they become trapped in the body, often resurfacing as physical symptoms or emotional imbalances. Feeling your feelings is one of the most direct paths to healing. It releases stored energy and breaks the cycle of repression.

HOW THIS LIFELINE SUPPORTS HEALING

- Disrupts patterns of emotional suppression and opens the door to integration and freedom
- Strengthens your connection to your inner truth and your capacity to express it
- Builds emotional resilience by helping you move through—not around—difficult feelings

One of the most transformative truths I've learned is this: feelings are meant to be felt.

They're not obstacles to avoid or problems to fix. They are invitations—guides—pointing us toward what needs to be seen, heard, and healed.

But I didn't always understand this. For much of my life, I feared difficult emotions. I tried to outrun them, numb them, or pretend they weren't there. What I eventually discovered was that the only way to truly heal is to feel.

When we allow emotions to surface and make space for them, we're not just honoring our experience—we're reclaiming the energy we've been using to resist. This softens fear and tension, making room for healing.

As Giten Tonkov writes in *Feel to Heal*:
"We can't selectively numb feelings. When we suppress one emotion, we limit our capacity to feel others—like joy, connection, and love."

The more I allowed myself to feel what was real, the more alive I became. Breathwork opened that door—gently, gradually, and with compassion.

THE FELT SENSE

One practice that helped me navigate emotional waves is the *Felt Sense*, a concept introduced by philosopher and psychotherapist Dr. Eugene Gendlin, creator of Focusing.

Gendlin teaches that transformation doesn't come from analyzing emotions, but from sensing them—feeling with the body, not thinking with the mind.

For example, when anxiety arises, I might notice tightness in my chest or buzzing in my arms. Instead of resisting, I tune in. I meet the sensation with presence, grounding myself in breath. This pairing—awareness and breath—is powerful. It allows emotions to shift and move without force.

Some emotions, like grief or rage, are physical in their intensity. In those moments, my breath becomes an anchor. It holds me steady as the storm passes. And when the wave moves through—as it always does—I'm left with more space, more softness.

THE ONLY WAY IS THROUGH

One of the deepest truths I've come to live by is this: the only way to release pain is to move through it.

We're often taught to avoid, distract, or numb ourselves when discomfort arises. But avoidance only prolongs suffering. What we resist, persists.

In the beginning, feeling everything was overwhelming. The emotional waves were massive. But over time, I learned to trust the process. Emotions are simply energy moving through the body—and meeting them allows that energy to flow and release.

What surprised me most? The more I stayed present in pain, the more my capacity for joy grew.

For so long, happiness felt distant. But as I let myself feel grief and fear, I found myself laughing more freely, loving more deeply. I wasn't outside of my life anymore—I was in it.

THE SCIENCE OF EMOTIONAL EXPRESSION

Feeling your feelings isn't just poetic—it's biological. Emotional energy lives not only in the mind, but in the body. When emotions are repressed, the nervous system bears the burden.

Dr. Bessel van der Kolk, author of *The Body Keeps the Score*, describes how unprocessed emotions are stored somatically—within muscles, fascia, posture, and breath patterns:
"Being able to feel safe with other people is probably the single

most important aspect of mental health. But safety begins inside your own body."

When emotions like grief, rage, or fear aren't given space, they remain unresolved. Over time, this internalized suppression can show up as chronic tension, fatigue, illness, or emotional numbing.

Feeling your feelings, on the other hand, activates the body's natural processing systems. Dr. Peter Levine, founder of *Somatic Experiencing*, explains that emotional energy must move through the body to complete its cycle. Allowing the body to feel and release reduces the likelihood of trauma becoming stuck.

Neuroscience supports this too. Emotional expression calms the amygdala (the brain's fear center) and increases regulation in the prefrontal cortex—the part responsible for insight, clarity, and decision-making.

Naming and feeling emotions also strengthens vagal tone, helping regulate the parasympathetic nervous system. This increases resilience, lowers stress, and enhances the ability to return to baseline after distress.

As Dr. Gabor Maté emphasizes:
"Emotions are not luxuries. They are the vital compass points of our life."

Feeling your feelings is not weakness—it's regulation. It's presence. It's how we metabolize life and reclaim our wholeness.

EMOTIONS ARE FLUID

One of the greatest gifts of emotional presence is the reminder that no feeling is final.

Emotions are like weather—temporary, shifting, alive. They are not flaws or failures. They are part of being human.

Feeling your feelings doesn't mean being ruled by them. In fact, it creates freedom. When we meet emotions as they are—without resistance—they loosen their grip. They move. We reclaim our power—not by controlling how we feel, but by allowing what's true to move through us.

This is the heart of healing: to meet what's real, moment by moment. In doing so, we return to our bodies, our hearts, and the wholeness we've carried all along.

REAL LIFE EXAMPLES OF FEEL ALL YOUR FEELINGS

- When frustration rises, instead of pushing it away, pause. Feel the heat, the tension in your chest—and let it be there without judgment. That presence creates space for release.
- A man going through a breakup has been avoiding his grief. One evening, he stops distracting himself and sits with the sadness. He lets the tears come. Afterward, he feels lighter. Healing has begun.
- A woman overwhelmed by anxiety and perfectionism feels pressure building. Instead of suppressing it, she pauses, breathes, and notices the tightness in her stomach. She allows herself to feel it—not to fix it, but simply to experience it. In that space, the anxiety begins to soften.

PRACTICE: EMOTIONAL CHECK-IN

Take a few quiet minutes each day to check in with yourself. This simple act of presence supports emotional flow and deepens self-awareness.

Find a comfortable seat and close your eyes. Take a few deep breaths.

Gently ask: How am I feeling right now? Let the answer arise without trying to fix or change it.

Notice where you feel it in your body—chest, stomach, jaw, shoulders.

Breathe into the sensation. Give it space.

When ready, exhale gently and imagine releasing the emotion from your body.

CHAPTER 11 | BEND–MOVE YOUR BODY AND LET IT MOVE YOU

Bend is the practice of moving your body in ways that feel nourishing, liberating, and alive. Whether it's yoga, walking, stretching, or dancing in your kitchen, movement clears emotional stagnation and reconnects you with your physical self.

Our bodies store tension—often emotional—and one of the most effective ways to release that energy is through intentional movement. Physical activity supports healing on every level: it lifts your mood, improves sleep, regulates your nervous system, and circulates vital life-force energy. Movement isn't just exercise—it's expression. It's embodiment. It's freedom.

HOW THIS LIFELINE SUPPORTS HEALING

- Releases stored trauma and emotional tension
- Boosts energy and mental clarity
- Builds resilience and strengthens the mind-body connection

Movement has long been a cornerstone of my emotional and physical well-being. I discovered running at sixteen, and it quickly became more than a workout—it was a lifeline. A daily reprieve from the chaos in my mind.

Growing up prone to anxiety, I now see how my body was trying to cope with deeper emotional wounds. I didn't have the language back then, but my instinctive pull toward movement was already guiding me toward healing. Running didn't just give me energy—it helped me process emotions I didn't yet know how to express.

With every stride, tension softened. Fog lifted. The endorphins rushing through me brought a sense of motivation and aliveness that had once felt out of reach. And it wasn't just the movement—it was the space: being outside, under the sky, in nature. There's something grounding about fresh air and open space that reconnects us to something bigger.

Over the years, movement has remained essential. When I slipped out of routine—during times of grief, burnout, or stress—I felt the difference almost immediately. My mind felt heavier. I became more emotionally reactive. Again and again, I've learned that movement isn't optional—it's vital. Not just for my body, but for my clarity, calm, and resilience.

THE SCIENCE OF MOVEMENT

The healing power of movement is well-documented. Physical activity releases endorphins, serotonin, and dopamine—feel-good brain chemicals that regulate mood, reduce stress, and support emotional well-being (Harvard Health, 2020). It also lowers cortisol, the stress hormone, restoring balance to the nervous system.

On a deeper level, movement reshapes the brain. Studies show that regular physical activity can increase the size of the hippocampus, the brain area linked to memory and emotional regulation (Erickson et al., 2011).

It also boosts neuroplasticity—your brain's ability to form new connections and adapt to change (Ratey, 2008). In other words, movement literally rewires us, strengthening our capacity to grow through and recover from emotional pain.

Trauma doesn't just live in our minds; it lives in our bodies. Somatic therapy reminds us that movement is one of the most powerful tools for physically processing and releasing what words cannot touch (Levine, 2010). Whether it's stretching, flowing, or even shaking, movement activates a natural release valve for built-up emotional energy. It's like the body saying, *"It's safe to let go now."*

RECONNECTING TO THE BODY

Even a gentle stretch or mindful walk can bring clarity. Movement reconnects us to our bodies—not as something to judge, but as a source of wisdom and strength. Over time, we become more attuned to how our bodies feel, deepening emotional awareness.

Adding breath to movement strengthens this connection. Conscious breathing during movement helps regulate the nervous system and supports emotional release. It's not about burning calories—it's about coming home to yourself, breath by breath.

Movement is a simple, accessible tool for healing. You don't need a gym. You don't need gear. Just a willingness to begin. Whether it's five minutes of stretching, a walk, or a wild dance in your living room—your body will thank you. And over time, so will your heart.

Like every healing practice, consistency matters. Start small. Move in ways that feel good, not forced. The more you move, the more you'll feel its quiet power—grounding you, freeing you, bringing you back to yourself. Healing doesn't always happen in stillness. Sometimes, it begins with a bend.

REAL LIFE EXAMPLES OF BEND

- After a painful breakup, a woman dances in her living room. As the music moves her, so does the grief—until it starts to release. Each session softens her pain and reconnects her to joy.
- A woman under chronic stress turns to yoga. Through daily movement and breath, she softens tension in her shoulders and back. The practice grounds her, offering peace and resilience.
- A man processing deep grief takes up rock climbing. As he climbs, the physical challenge gives his mind a break and his body a purpose. Each reach mirrors his inner journey—showing him he is strong enough to keep going.

PRACTICE: DAILY FLOW OF MOVEMENT

Set aside 10–15 minutes each day for intentional movement. This could be stretching, yoga, a walk, or freeform dancing.

Tune in: How does your body feel? Where is there tension or stiffness?

Move slowly and intuitively—let your body guide you rather than following a set routine. Allow the movement to express the energy you're holding, whether slow and fluid or fast and full of release.

Breathe deeply throughout. Notice how movement and breath together create space—for your emotions, your body, and your healing.

CHAPTER 12 | BREATHE—COME BACK TO YOUR SENSES

THE BRIDGE BETWEEN MIND AND BODY

As we've explored throughout this book, breathwork is a conscious, intentional practice of using the breath to influence the body, mind, and emotions. The breath is the bridge between the conscious and unconscious. Through mindful breathing, we access deeper layers of the psyche, release stored emotions, and soothe the nervous system.

Breathing is unique—it's both automatic and voluntary. This dual nature allows us to shift our emotional and physical state in real time. Breathwork activates the parasympathetic nervous system, reducing anxiety, promoting relaxation, and releasing trauma held in the body. For those who feel disconnected from themselves or live in a constant state of stress, the breath becomes a way to come home—to calm, to presence, to yourself.

HOW THIS LIFELINE SUPPORTS HEALING

- Resets the nervous system, shifting you from stress to relaxation
- Unlocks deeply held emotional tension for release and healing

- Anchors you in the present moment, enhancing mindfulness and grounding

Breathing is something we do all day, every day, without thinking. But your breath is also one of the most powerful tools you have for healing, grounding, and transformation.

When I began my healing journey, I didn't fully appreciate its significance. I knew how physical exercise could ease anxiety, but breathwork offered something deeper—it met me in the stillness. In moments of overwhelm—fear, sadness, or grief—I turned to my breath. And each time, it brought me back to calm. It brought me back to my center.

BREATH AS AN ANCHOR

Mindful breathing became my anchor in the storm. Not just a way to calm my nervous system, but a way to reconnect with myself when I needed it the most.

When I allowed myself to simply breathe—fully, consciously—I didn't just feel air moving through my lungs. I felt my body soften, my mind quiet, and something deep within begin to settle. The breath held me when words couldn't.

THE SCIENCE OF BREATH

The breath is more than air—it's a built-in tool for nervous system regulation and emotional healing.

When we breathe slowly and intentionally, we stimulate the vagus nerve, activating the parasympathetic nervous system—the body's natural relaxation response (Porges, 2011). This lowers heart rate, reduces blood pressure, and brings the body into a state of calm.

Conversely, rapid, shallow breathing (often a stress response) engages the sympathetic nervous system, triggering fight-or-flight. Over time, this dysregulation can contribute to anxiety, emotional reactivity, and chronic health conditions.

As Drs. Patricia Gerbarg and Richard Brown write in *The Healing Power of the Breath*,
"By changing the patterns of breathing, we can change the patterns of our emotions."

Breathwork also helps regulate brainwave activity, shifting us from heightened beta states (stress, overthinking) into alpha or theta states, which support calm, creativity, and presence (Gerbarg & Brown, 2012).

James Nestor, author of *Breath*, explains how slow, nasal, rhythmic breathing supports lung capacity, cardiovascular health, and emotional stability.

Even a few minutes of conscious breath each day strengthens vagal tone, enhances resilience, and improves emotional flexibility. Because the breath is always available, it's one of the most empowering tools we have—no equipment, no cost, no permission required.

Dr. Andrew Huberman, neuroscientist at Stanford, shares, *"Physiological sighs—a double inhale followed by a long exhale—are one of the fastest ways to shift from stress to calm."*

The breath is a regulator, a releaser, and a reminder that healing can happen moment by moment—starting with something as simple as a conscious exhale.

REAL LIFE EXAMPLES OF BREATHE

- After trauma, a woman uses breathwork to manage anxiety. During panic, she practices box breathing and feels her body shift from tension to calm. Over time, it becomes her go-to tool for emotional stability.
- A man balancing a demanding job and family notices stress building throughout the day. He pauses, places a hand on his belly, and takes slow, intentional breaths. As he exhales,

he visualizes releasing the weight of his responsibilities. This simple practice restores clarity and calm.

- A college student struggles with performance anxiety. The night before a big exam, panic sets in. Instead of spiraling, she practices 4-7-8 breathing: inhale for 4, hold for 7, exhale for 8. After a few minutes, her body relaxes, her thoughts settle, and she feels ready to face the challenge with steadiness.

PRACTICE: GROUNDING BREATHWORK FOR CALM AND CLARITY

Set aside 5–10 minutes each day for this grounding practice.

Find a comfortable seat—on the floor or in a chair. Sit tall with a straight spine.

Close your eyes and take a few slow, deep breaths. Let your belly rise as you inhale, fall gently as you exhale.

Begin box breathing:

- *Inhale for a count of 4*
- *Hold for a count of 4*
- *Exhale for a count of 4*
- *Hold for a count of 4*
- *Repeat for several cycles, letting the rhythm guide you*

With each inhale, draw in calm and clarity. With each exhale, release stress and tension.

Feel your body grounding into the present moment. Let this practice reset your nervous system—a space for body and mind to soften, release, and heal.

CHAPTER 13 | SOUND–LISTEN DEEPLY, EXPRESS FREELY

Sound, in all its forms, holds profound healing power. Whether you're listening to music, singing, drumming, humming, or immersing yourself in sound frequencies, sound is a lifeline that can shift emotional states and recalibrate the nervous system.

Across cultures and centuries, sound has been used as a tool for healing. Its vibrations influence brainwaves, helping us move from stress and anxiety into states of relaxation, presence, and peace.

Music, in particular, has a unique ability to access emotions that words alone cannot reach. Through sound, we connect to something larger than ourselves—something that transcends logic and speaks directly to the soul.

HOW THIS LIFELINE SUPPORTS HEALING

- Instantly shifts emotional and mental states—from agitation to calm\
- Grounds us in the present moment, helping release past trauma and anxiety

- Opens pathways for emotional expression and the release of stuck energy
- Uses vibration to stimulate the body and clear energetic blockages

RESONANCE AND REPAIR

Sound became an unexpected but essential companion in my own experience. At first, it was background noise—pleasant, but passive. Over time, music became part of the process itself. I began creating playlists based on how I felt or what I needed—whether to reconnect, reflect, or release.

Certain songs resonated like mantras, unlocking emotions and memories I hadn't realized I was still carrying. Humming or softly singing along became ritual. What began as instinctive turned into something deeply intentional.

Unbeknownst to me at the time, humming and singing were stimulating my vagus nerve—a key player in regulating emotional and physiological balance. Through sound, I was inviting calm, presence, and emotional release.

Eventually, I began to create sound, not just consume it. I tapped my hands or feet during breathwork to sync rhythm with my breath. I introduced a simple drum—not to perform music, but to express what words couldn't.

Drumming, humming, and gentle vocalizing became tools for emotional processing and presence.

Sound bypasses the thinking mind and communicates directly with the body. In moments of grief, sadness, or frustration, sound became a quiet force that helped me move through emotion rather than around it.

THE SCIENCE OF SOUND

Sound healing isn't just a poetic idea—it's backed by growing scientific evidence. Specific sound frequencies, like binaural beats, can regulate brain activity, guiding us into states of calm, focus, and meditation (Le Scouarnec et al., 2001).

Sound shifts brainwave frequencies, directly influencing mental and emotional states:

Alpha waves promote relaxation

Beta waves sharpen focus

Theta waves support meditation and dreaming

Delta waves bring deep rest (Mason et al., 2007)

On a cellular level, sound acts as a vibrational force, helping break up emotional and energetic blockages (Goldsby et al., 2017). Intense emotions—trauma, grief, or frustration—often get stored in the body, and sound can help move and release them.

In my own experience, sound became especially powerful when paired with breathwork. Humming during exhale or tapping a rhythm during a breath session helped me access stored emotions that needed release.

The combination of sound and breath opened a pathway to peace, regulation, and inner clarity—a deeply grounding experience.

REAL LIFE EXAMPLES OF SOUND

- A woman navigating a high-stress job listens to nature sounds—ocean waves, birdsong—while working. The sound brings peace amidst the chaos. Over time, she pairs it with deep breathing, creating a grounding ritual that helps her stay centered.
- A man coping with anxiety uses binaural beats to relax before meetings or stressful deadlines. The rhythmic tones slow his heart rate and calm his mind. With practice, he learns to shift

into relaxation on demand, using sound as a reliable tool for emotional regulation.

- A woman feeling isolated begins chanting affirmations softly. At first, it feels unfamiliar, but gradually she grows confident in her voice. She starts singing the words, feeling their power resonate in her chest. Vocalizing becomes a form of self-connection, helping her rewrite her inner dialogue and reclaim her sense of agency.

PRACTICE: SOUND IMMERSION FOR EMOTIONAL BALANCE

Set aside 10–15 minutes each day to engage with sound in a way that feels nourishing and expressive. This could be listening to calming music, humming a melody, drumming, or singing

Sit comfortably and close your eyes.

Tune into the vibration of the sound—let it wash over you and move through your body.

Notice what emotions or sensations arise. Do certain sounds bring tension or memories? Does something inside you begin to soften?

Explore sound healing frequencies—binaural beats or Tibetan singing bowls—to deepen the experience.

Let this time be about tuning in, feeling, and expressing. Allow sound to guide you into emotional recalibration, bringing your nervous system back into harmony.

CHAPTER 14 | CIRCLE–BE HELD, HOLD OTHERS

Circle refers to the healing power of community. It's about being seen, supported, and held by others who understand and witness you on your healing journey. As human beings, we are wired for connection, and the quality of our relationships profoundly impacts our emotional and physical well-being.

Isolation is one of the greatest challenges during times of pain. It reinforces the illusion that we are alone in our suffering and can fuel feelings of shame and unworthiness. Community counters that isolation. It reminds us we are not alone, that our experiences matter, and that we are deserving of love and support.

Being witnessed—genuinely seen and heard—can be as healing as any inner work. The energy of a compassionate group amplifies that healing.

HOW THIS LIFELINE SUPPORTS HEALING

- Connection breaks the isolation that often accompanies trauma
- Being witnessed provides validation, encouragement, and emotional regulation

- Shared experience fosters empathy and reminds us we are not alone

WHERE BELONGING BEGINS

Before the drugging, I felt grounded within my large, extended family. While the dynamics weren't always easy, those relationships offered a sense of safety and belonging. Even before everything unraveled, subtle shifts began—certain connections became strained or distant. The warmth I once depended on quietly faded, and that alone carried its own grief.

When everything collapsed, I reached for familiar support systems—family, friends, institutions—but they felt out of reach. The isolation was devastating. Yet in that silence, something else began to form. Without the usual scaffolding, I turned inward—and discovered a steadiness I hadn't known before.

Then, something surprising happened: new connections emerged. In unexpected places, I found spaces where healing was the shared intention, and vulnerability was welcomed. These were not just friendships—they were lifelines. People showed up with presence, not pity. They listened with openness, not judgment. They reminded me that I didn't have to heal alone.

The people we surround ourselves with influence our healing in profound ways. Our closest relationships can either reinforce our pain or reflect our potential. That's why it's important to be intentional about the company we keep—not just kind people, but those whose lives inspire us to grow.

As I healed, my circle shifted. Some people remained—steadfast and loving through the storm. Others drifted away, and though their absence stung, it also brought clarity. I began to see who was truly aligned with the woman I was becoming.

Today, my relationships are grounded in authenticity and mutual respect. The refining of my inner circle became part of the healing itself. True community isn't about numbers—it's about depth. When you are seen in your wholeness, held in your truth, and loved without condition, healing doesn't just accelerate—it deepens.

THE SCIENCE OF CONNECTION

Connection isn't just an emotional experience—it's a biological one. Human beings are wired for relationship, and meaningful connection has a measurable impact on health and well-being.

When we feel safe and supported, our bodies release oxytocin, often called the "bonding hormone" or "love hormone." As Dr. Sue Carter explains, oxytocin strengthens emotional bonds, reduces anxiety, and helps regulate the nervous system. It's one reason we feel calmer in the presence of someone we trust.

On the flip side, isolation activates our stress response. Chronic loneliness is linked to elevated cortisol levels, which contribute to inflammation, sleep disturbances, and reduced immune function (Heinrichs et al., 2003).

In contrast, people with strong social ties tend to recover more quickly from illness, manage stress more effectively, and experience greater resilience.

As Dr. Dan Siegel writes:

"Connection creates integration. Integration creates resilience."

Being seen and known by others provides psychological oxygen. It validates our inner world and co-regulates our nervous system—meaning, being near someone calm and empathetic can help bring us back into balance. In trauma healing spaces, this is known as co-regulation: the soothing of one nervous system through safe connection with another. Community helps us heal not just emotionally, but physiologically.

Belonging also strengthens identity and meaning. In a compassionate circle, we internalize: *I matter. I'm not alone. I am enough.* Rebuilding my own support circle didn't just restore emotional stability—it gave me a renewed sense of wholeness. Research and lived experience show: we are not meant to heal in isolation. We are wired to heal together.

REAL LIFE EXAMPLES OF CIRCLE\

- A man navigating sobriety joins a recovery group. As he listens to others' stories, he finds courage to share his own. The group offers camaraderie, accountability, and hope. The collective journey reminds him he's not alone—and that healing is possible, one step at a time.
- A woman new to yoga feels unsure and intimidated. Over time, she bonds with a small group of fellow practitioners. They support each other, share tips, and connect beyond the mat. Through their encouragement, she gains confidence, realizing growth is magnified in the presence of community.
- A person grieving a deep loss joins an online support group. At first, they hesitate to share—but reading others' stories brings unexpected comfort. When they finally speak, they're met with empathy and understanding. The space becomes a container for healing, showing them that even in grief, they are not alone.

PRACTICE: CONNECT WITH YOUR PEOPLE

Each week, choose one intentional way to connect with your community. Join a support group, attend a class (in person or online), or reach out to a trusted friend for a heart-centered conversation.

Allow yourself to be seen—no masks, no filters. Share something real. And just as importantly, practice active listening. Hold space for others with the same compassion you long to receive.

If you don't yet have a community, take one small step to create it. Invite a few kindred spirits to gather regularly. Explore spaces—virtual or local—where authenticity and vulnerability are honored.

Your circle doesn't need to be large. It just needs to be real. When we show up authentically, we open the door to true connection—and healing becomes a shared experience.

CHAPTER 15 | EXPRESS—LET YOUR TRUTH BE SEEN

Expression and creation are powerful outlets through which we release emotion, speak our truth, and transform pain into beauty. Whether through art, writing, dance, or another creative medium, self-expression allows us to bypass logic and language, communicating directly from the soul.

Creativity grants access to parts of ourselves that words alone often can't reach. When we create, we enter a state of "flow"—an immersive awareness that brings clarity, peace, and presence. In that space, we become both witness and participant in our healing, allowing emotions to rise, move, and transform.

HOW THIS LIFELINE SUPPORTS HEALING

- Creativity allows for the release of emotions that may be hard to articulate
- It provides a safe outlet for exploring your inner world
- The act of creating fosters empowerment, purpose, and self-trust

FINDING MY VOICE

Telling my story wasn't just about seeking justice or sharing my experience—it was a primal need to release the weight of trauma. Long before I could name what had happened, I was recording voice memos: raw, unfiltered fragments of thought and emotion. These early expressions were private and messy—but they were mine. They marked the beginning of externalizing pain I instinctively knew I couldn't carry alone.

When I finally grasped the full magnitude of what I'd endured—and the institutional failure that followed—I turned to the only platform that felt accessible: social media. It wasn't strategic. It was survival. I needed to be heard. I needed to speak into the silence.

What began as a desperate act of expression quickly evolved. Though my words were sometimes misunderstood—or even used against me—they also resonated. People listened. Some saw their own pain reflected in mine. Others offered solidarity. In that vulnerable act of sharing, I found connection. And in connection, I began to heal.

RETURN TO BLISS

Around this time, I returned to a long-forgotten love: photography. I'd always meant to come back to it when life felt less demanding. But healing rarely waits for the perfect moment.

As I walked through grief and confusion, my camera became more than a tool—it became a companion. Like when I was a teenager in the darkroom, I found comfort in noticing light, shadow, and stillness. But now, I wasn't just capturing what I saw—I was capturing how I felt. Grief. Wonder. Hope.

Photography became meditation. It grounded me, helped me notice beauty again, and gently reconnected me to myself. Through the lens, I found my joy. I remembered peace.

THE NEUROSCIENCE OF CREATIVITY

This wasn't just emotional—it was biological. Engaging in creative activities like writing, painting, or music releases dopamine—the natural "feel-good" chemical that lifts mood, boosts motivation, and builds resilience. It's like a built-in antidepressant, helping us feel more alive and hopeful (Levitin, 2019).

Creativity also lights up the prefrontal cortex, the brain's executive center responsible for emotional regulation and decision-making—areas often impacted by trauma. By engaging in creative expression, we forge new neural pathways and help release emotions that might be stuck beneath the surface (Dietrich, 2004).

For me, when words failed, photography became my language. Often, I didn't fully understand what I was feeling until I saw it reflected in an image. Visual storytelling held space for *all the feelings*, without needing explanation or judgment. It became a quiet conversation between my inner and outer worlds.

Creative expression is not only therapeutic—it's sacred. It reconnects us to the vibrant, joyful parts of ourselves that trauma can obscure. We remember that we are not defined by what happened to us, but by what we create in response.

This very book is an act of expression. Writing it has helped me make sense of the intangible, integrate the pain, and offer something meaningful to others. It's a reminder that our stories matter. And when we express them, we invite transformation—for ourselves and for those who witness us.

REAL LIFE EXAMPLES OF EXPRESS

- A woman healing childhood trauma begins journaling. At first, her words are private and raw. Eventually, she writes poetry—her truth in verse. As she shares her work, she finds empowerment in expressing herself and connection with others who recognize their own stories in hers.

- A man battling anxiety takes up guitar. At first, his music is chaotic, echoing his inner turmoil. But with time, it softens and evolves. He begins writing songs, turning tension into rhythm. Music becomes a lifeline, helping him express what he can't always say.
- A woman grappling with self-doubt picks up a camera. She starts with landscapes, then moves to self-portraits. Slowly, she sees herself differently—through a lens of compassion. Photography helps her reframe her story, find beauty in her imperfections, and reclaim her power.

PRACTICE: CREATIVE EXPRESSION

Set aside 20 minutes each day for a creative practice that speaks to you—writing, dancing, painting, crafting, or music. Let go of outcomes. This is about process, not perfection.

Start with a few deep breaths to ground yourself. Let your emotions rise. Then create—without judgment, without filter. Let colors, sounds, or shapes say what words can't.

Afterwards, reflect: Has anything shifted? Over time, this practice creates space for healing, helping emotions flow and transform into beauty.

CHAPTER 16 | HEART & HANDS– SERVICE, GRATITUDE, AND TRUST

Heart & Hands is the practice of living from love. It means serving others from a place of fullness, not depletion. It means leading with gratitude, not grasping. And it means offering your energy to the world with humility and grace.

This lifeline is about what we give—and how we give it. It's about bringing our whole selves to the moment, whether we're offering care, making dinner, saying thank you, or trusting something bigger than ourselves. Our hearts guide our intention. Our hands make it real.

HOW THIS LIFELINE SUPPORTS HEALING

- Anchors us in gratitude and presence
- Transforms powerlessness into purpose
- Builds trust in life through small acts of service and surrender

RETURNING TO LOVE

During the darkest parts of my journey, I felt stripped bare. So much had been taken from me—certainty, connection, identity. I clung to whatever sense of control I could grasp. But eventually, control became its own prison. What I needed wasn't more control—it was more trust.

One morning, feeling especially hollow, I stood by the window with a cup of coffee in my hands. Outside, the light settled over the hillside. The trees moved in the breeze. Something about the quiet beauty stirred something in me—a reminder that even in the heaviness, there was still something to be thankful for.

I had been so focused on surviving that I had stopped seeing what was right in front of me. That morning marked the return to this lifeline. I began naming the good. Out loud. Every day.

"I'm grateful for my home. For the trees. For this breath."

That practice changed everything. I started asking: What can I give today? Not because I had to, but because I wanted to feel connected again—to something greater than my story.

When I began showing up for others—through kindness, service, presence—I found parts of myself returning. I didn't need to fix anyone. I didn't need to be perfect. I just needed to love well.

GRATITUDE AS REORIENTATION

Gratitude isn't just a mood booster—it's a lens shift. It's the practice of anchoring into what is working, what is here, what is real.

In the midst of confusion or heartbreak, gratitude reminded me: There is still beauty. There is still good.

It helped me orient toward love—especially when fear or scarcity threatened to take over. Rather than demanding that life meet me perfectly, I began to notice what life was already offering. I thanked the breath. I thanked the stillness. I thanked the chance to keep going.

Some days, my list was short. Some days, I didn't feel like it. But over time, gratitude softened the edges of my pain and reconnected me to possibility.

THE SCIENCE OF GRATITUDE, SERVICE AND TRUST

Research shows that gratitude, service, and trust are not only spiritually enriching—they're biologically and psychologically regulating.

Gratitude practices have been linked to increased happiness, reduced anxiety, and improved sleep. In a landmark study, Dr. Robert Emmons and Dr. Michael McCullough found that people who kept daily gratitude journals reported significantly greater optimism and well-being—even weeks after the practice ended.

Gratitude also lowers cortisol and activates brain regions associated with empathy and reward, such as the prefrontal cortex (Zahn et al., 2009). This shift supports nervous system regulation, reinforcing a sense of inner safety and presence.

Trust plays a similar role. According to psychologist Kelly McGonigal, cultivating trust reduces the physiological effects of stress. When we choose trust—even in small ways—we increase oxytocin levels and strengthen our capacity for emotional resilience.

As Dr. David DeSteno writes in Emotional Success:

"Gratitude, compassion, and pride—when cultivated intentionally—make us more honest, generous, and trustworthy."

Service, too, has measurable benefits. Acts of generosity trigger the release of dopamine and endorphins, boosting mood and creating what researchers call the "helper's high." These acts also shift attention away from personal struggle, activating a sense of purpose and connection that is deeply regulating.

A study by Crum, Salovey, and Achor (2013) found that participants who viewed their daily work as service—no matter the task—experienced lower burnout and higher job satisfaction. It wasn't about what they did. It was about the intention behind it.

When we orient toward gratitude, trust, and service, we move out of fear and into presence. We shift from contraction to expansion, from isolation to interconnection. These aren't grand gestures—they're quiet rewirings. And over time, they become a powerful foundation for healing.

WHAT YOU OFFER MATTERS

You don't need to volunteer at a shelter or start a nonprofit to live with Heart & Hands. Service is the way you smile at a stranger. The way you listen without fixing. The way you pray for someone silently.

It's the presence you bring to the room. The energy you offer through your actions.

During my own journey, I often felt like I had nothing left to give. But when I shifted the question from How can I be useful? to How can I be present?—something opened.

Even small offerings—like cooking a meal for a friend, holding a door for a stranger, or leaving a voice note for a loved one—felt sacred. Because it wasn't about productivity. It was about presence. About letting love move through me, however it could.

REAL LIFE EXAMPLES OF HEART & HANDS

- A woman going through a divorce feels emotionally raw and uncertain. Instead of withdrawing completely, she offers to cook dinner for a neighbor who's had surgery. In doing so, she feels useful again—and less alone in her own pain.
- A young man navigating depression begins a simple practice: each morning, he writes down three things he's grateful for.

Some days, it's just coffee and sunlight. But over time, he notices a subtle shift. His world feels less dark. His capacity for hope grows.

- A parent struggling with anxiety begins using breathwork before bedtime, placing a hand on her heart and silently offering gratitude for her children. She does it even on hard days—especially on hard days. That small moment of connection helps her reenter the next day with grace.

PRACTICE: A HEART & HANDS RITUAL

Each day, ask yourself:

What can I give today?

What can I appreciate today?

What can I trust today?

Keep it simple—one word or phrase is enough to set your focus.

CHAPTER 17 | BODY TEMPLE–CARE FOR THE VESSEL THAT CARRIES YOU

The *Body Temple* represents the sacred act of honoring and caring for our physical selves. Our bodies are the vessels through which we experience life, and how we tend to them shapes our emotional, mental, and spiritual well-being.

This isn't about chasing perfection or aesthetics—it's about cultivating vitality, balance, and presence. When we nourish our bodies, we anchor ourselves in the moment. When we rest, we restore clarity. When we move, we shift energy and build resilience. These everyday acts of care become the scaffolding for healing and wholeness.

HOW THIS LIFELINE SUPPORTS HEALING

- Movement and nutrition boost feel-good chemicals like serotonin and endorphins
- Sleep supports emotional stability and stress resilience
- Consistent self-care strengthens self-trust and embodiment

THE BODY AS SACRED GROUND

Learning to treat my body as sacred was a profound shift. It meant moving from criticism to compassion, from neglect to nurturance. I began to understand that physical health wasn't just a bonus—it was foundational.

Whenever I felt off—depleted, anxious, or overwhelmed—I could almost always trace it back to how I was (or wasn't) caring for my body.

Simple things—eating nourishing food, getting enough sleep, hydrating, and moving—became quiet but powerful acts of reclamation. They weren't glamorous or dramatic. They were steady. Loving. Vital.

NUTRITION: FUELING YOUR INNER STRENGTH

What we eat doesn't just shape our bodies—it shapes our mood, clarity, and capacity to cope. The gut-brain connection is real, as Dr. Emeran Mayer's research confirms.

When I shifted to more whole foods—leafy greens, healthy fats, clean proteins—it wasn't about rules or restriction. It was about asking: *Does this nourish me?* My body always knew. I just had to start listening.

HYDRATION; THE UNSUNG HERO

Water became one of the most potent forms of care in my daily rhythm. Research shows that even mild dehydration can mimic symptoms of anxiety and fatigue. Sipping water became more than a habit—it became a ritual. A pause. A soft reminder: *You are worthy of tending.*

Healing isn't always loud. Sometimes it's in the quiet of pouring a glass of water and taking a long, mindful sip.

SLEEP: A RADICAL ACT OF REGULATION

Sleep is sacred. As Matthew Walker shares in *Why We Sleep*, it's essential for emotional regulation, memory, and resilience.

When I created a gentle nighttime rhythm—dim lights, no screens, soft music, a little breathwork—everything changed. My nervous system found rhythm again. Sleep became more than rest. It became restoration.

Choosing sleep became a form of rebellion against burnout—a return to trusting the wisdom of my body.

MINDFUL MODERATION: HONORING THE BODY'S INNER COMPASS

So many of our habits are driven by unconscious seeking—comfort, escape, regulation. Instead of judging those habits, I got curious.

I asked: *Does this soothe me or numb me? Does it connect me to myself or distract me?*

That shift—toward awareness without shame—transformed everything. It let me practice care, not control. And with that, trust returned.

THE SCIENCE OF CARING FOR THE BODY

Tending to your body isn't just helpful—it's healing at the physiological level.

Nutrition directly affects emotional well-being. The gut and brain are connected through the vagus nerve and neurotransmitters. Inflammation and poor digestion can contribute to anxiety and mood disorders. Eating whole, nutrient-rich foods supports emotional balance and cognitive clarity (Mayer, *The Mind-Gut Connection*).

Hydration is equally essential. Even a 1–2% drop in hydration can impair mood, focus, and energy levels (Popkin et al., 2010). Water supports digestion, temperature regulation, and emotional stability.

Sleep is perhaps the most underrated healing tool. Deep sleep helps process emotions, reset cortisol levels, and enhance empathy and calm (Walker, *Why We Sleep*). Lack of sleep amplifies fear responses and reduces self-regulation.

Movement releases endorphins and boosts serotonin and dopamine. It improves memory, lowers stress, and clears emotional stagnation from the body.

Together, these foundational elements—food, water, rest, and movement—create a resilient internal ecosystem. Caring for your body supports your nervous system, enabling it to regulate, recover, and thrive.

A BLUEPRINT FOR THRIVING

Caring for the body isn't separate from healing—it is healing.

Our physical vessel holds the emotions, memories, and sensations we're working through. When we care for it intentionally, we create space for clarity, strength, and ease.

The simple things—eating well, moving, resting, hydrating—aren't just healthy habits. They're declarations: *I matter. I'm worth caring for.*

These small, daily acts become a foundation we can return to—again and again.

REAL LIFE EXAMPLES OF BODY TEMPLE

- A woman healing from anxiety begins a nightly ritual: screens off by 9 p.m., soft music, and deep breathing. As her sleep improves, her nervous system calms. Morning walks follow. Slowly, her anxiety eases, and clarity returns.

- A man recovering from burnout starts cooking for himself and drinking more water. He cuts back on caffeine and adds light strength workouts. His energy grows—and with it, his capacity to handle stress. His body becomes his ally again.
- After a long illness, a woman begins with gentle yoga and slowly shifts to more movement and whole foods. Each week brings more strength and balance. Her physical healing deepens her emotional resilience. She remembers: transformation begins with care.

PRACTICE: SIMPLE AND CONSISTENT ADDS UP

Design a simple, sustainable daily routine that supports your physical well-being. Start small:

> Take a 30-minute walk
>
> Prepare a nourishing meal
>
> Go to bed at the same time each night
>
> Drink a full glass of water when you wake up

Build slowly. Listen to your body. Let this become a rhythm of support—not pressure. Over time, these small steps become a foundation of strength that can carry you through anything.

PRACTICE MAKES PROGRESS

Healing doesn't always arrive in a moment of revelation. Often, it arrives quietly—through a breath you take, a hand you place on your heart, a small act of kindness, or the soft acknowledgment of a feeling you didn't know you could hold.

These nine Lifelines—Radical Self-Love, Feel All Your Feelings, Bend, Breathe, Sound, Circle, Express, Heart & Hands, and Body Temple—are your companions on that journey. They are not just practices; they are ways of returning to yourself again and again.

I didn't show up for all of them every day. Some days, I forgot. Some days, old habits whispered louder than intention. And yet, the moments I did—when I paused to notice my breath, when I moved my body even for five minutes, when I offered a kind word or an act of presence—those were the moments that built the scaffolding for everything else.

INTEGRATION INTO DAILY LIFE

The Lifelines aren't about perfection. They are invitations. Gentle ways to return to your center, to remember who you are beneath fear, grief, or exhaustion. You don't need a perfect schedule, a fancy ritual, or hours of uninterrupted time. Start small. Five deep breaths. A stretch. A note of gratitude. A song you hum aloud. A moment of presence with a friend. These tiny acts ripple outward—they compound.

Imagine your day as a series of small touch points:

- Morning: Place a hand on your heart. Speak a kind phrase to yourself. Breathe. Anchor into presence.
- Midday: Move. Walk, stretch, dance. Notice your emotions. Let them flow. Create. Listen. Connect. Even a brief check-in with a friend can recalibrate your nervous system.
- Evening: Nourish your body with food and water. Rest. Reflect. Let gratitude and service guide the closing of your day.

REFLECTION PROMPT

Which Lifeline calls to you today?
What is one small, real action you could take to honor it?

Let it be simple.

Let it be real.

Let it be yours.

With presence, with trust, with love—you return.

PART FOUR | FROM AIR TO EMBODIMENT: A GUIDE TO BREATHWORK PRACTICES

"The body always leads us home... if we can simply learn to trust its language."

— Rochelle Schieck

In the previous section, we explored the Lifelines—the foundational practices that shaped my healing journey. Breathwork was not just one of those Lifelines; it was the thread that wove them all together. It was the practice that connected mind, body, and heart, offering a tangible way to return to presence, process emotion, and reclaim calm.

Now, we move from understanding to application. This section invites you to experience the breath as I did—not just as theory, but as a living, embodied practice. Here, you'll find accessible tools to help you regulate your nervous system, ground into your body, release stuck energy and emotion, and reconnect with your inner resilience—one breath at a time.

These practices are meant to meet you where you are, whether you have five minutes or twenty. They are not about doing it "right," but about returning to yourself through the simple, transformative power of your own breath.

KNOW BEFORE YOU BREATHE: GENERAL GUIDANCE, HEALTH CONSIDERATIONS AND CONTRAINDICATIONS

Before we explore the breathing techniques in the next section, it's important to pause and review some key guidelines and health considerations. While breathwork can be a powerful tool for healing and transformation, it's essential to approach it with mindfulness and care.

TAKE IT SLOW
Begin with shorter sessions, especially if you're new to breathwork. Gradually increase the duration and intensity as you become more familiar with the techniques.

CREATE A SAFE SPACE
Ensure you have a quiet, comfortable environment to practice in, free from distractions. This helps maximize the benefits and allows for a deeper connection to the practice.

LISTEN TO YOUR BODY

Pay attention to how your body is responding during the exercises. If you feel lightheaded, dizzy, or uncomfortable, slow down or stop. Breathwork should feel empowering, not overwhelming.

STAY PRESENT

This practice works best when you are fully present. Focus on your breath and any sensations that arise in your body. Allow thoughts or emotions to surface without judgment.

Breathwork is generally safe and supportive for most people, but certain practices—such as Breath Holds, Conscious Connected Breath, and Breath of Fire—can place additional demands on the body. If you have any underlying health conditions, it's important to proceed with care.

Your well-being is the priority. Breathwork should always feel supportive, never forced or overwhelming. Begin gently, listen to your body, and honor its signals. This is a personal journey—there's no rush.

If you live with any of the following conditions, please consult your healthcare provider before engaging in the above-mentioned breathwork styles:

MEDICAL/PHYSICAL CONDITIONS

- Cardiovascular issues
    - High blood pressure (uncontrolled)
    - Coronary artery disease
    - History of heart attacks
    - Irregular heartbeat or arrhythmias
- Respiratory conditions
    - Asthma (unless well-managed and with inhaler on hand)

- COPD (Chronic Obstructive Pulmonary Disease)
            - Severe lung disease
    - Seizure disorders
        - Epilepsy
        - History of seizures (especially without medication or control)
    - Pregnancy
        - Particularly in the first and third trimesters, unless under guidance of a trained prenatal breathwork facilitator
    - Recent surgeries or injuries
        - Especially abdominal, heart, brain, or lung surgeries
        - Broken bones, spinal injuries, or significant muscular strain
    - Glaucoma or retinal detachment
    - Aneurysms
        - Or family history of brain aneurysms
    - Severe migraines
        - Breath practices can sometimes intensify symptoms
    - Blood clotting disorders
        - Or those on blood thinners

MENTAL HEALTH CONSIDERATIONS
- Schizophrenia
- Bipolar disorder (especially manic phases)
- Severe PTSD
    - May be retraumatizing if not held in a safe, trauma-informed container
- Dissociative disorders

- Unstable psychiatric conditions
- History of psychosis or delusions
- Recent trauma
    - Especially if not yet integrated or supported by professional therapy

Substance Abuse

- Currently under the influence of alcohol or drugs
- Detoxing or in acute withdrawal from substances
    - Especially without medical support

RELATIVE CONTRAINDICATIONS (USE WITH CAUTION OR PROFESSIONAL GUIDANCE):

- Anxiety or panic disorders
    - May cause hyperventilation if not guided gently
- Depression
- Chronic fatigue or adrenal insufficiency
- Complex trauma or history of emotional suppression
- People new to breathwork or with no prior somatic experience

Best Practices for Safety

- Always check with a medical or mental health professional if uncertain.
- For anyone with health concerns, a gentler breath style such as:
    - Coherent Breathing (5–6 breaths/min)
    - Box Breathing
    - 4-7-8 Breathing
    - Breath Awareness

In addition, if you have a history of sexual trauma, complex trauma, or other unprocessed emotional experiences, please know that certain breathwork practices may surface intense sensations or emotions. This is not unusual—breathwork can open the door to deep release and healing. However, it's essential that you feel safe and resourced.

You may benefit from practicing alongside a trauma-informed breathwork facilitator, coach, or therapist who can help you navigate any strong responses with compassion and care. Always go at your own pace. You're in charge of your experience, and there's nothing to prove or push through.

PRACTICE, NOT PERFECTION

As mentioned earlier, there are countless breathwork modalities—from ancient yogic pranayama to modern methods like Wim Hof. The techniques I share here aren't meant to be comprehensive. They're simply the ones I turned to most often; the ones that created meaningful shifts for me. If you discover a different style that resonates more deeply, trust that. Your journey is your own, and your intuition remains one of your greatest guides.

To support this journey, I've included a list of books and resources that have deeply influenced my own healing and breathwork practice. With breathwork's growing presence in western culture, there's no shortage of materials—books, podcasts, videos, and courses—to help you deepen your exploration. But no matter what you choose, your most powerful tool will always be your presence. The practice that works best is the one you return to consistently—with curiosity, openness, and compassion.

The next section is your invitation into the breath itself—not just to read about it, but to feel it, to try it, and to experience how it moves through your own body. These guided practices are meant to be simple, adaptable, and repeatable. Let this be your return-to guide—something you revisit again and again, whether you're grounding in a moment of stress, reconnecting after disconnection, or simply carving out space to breathe with intention.

And now, let's begin.

CHAPTER 18 | BREATHING WITH ATTENTION

Breath awareness is the most foundational—and accessible—form of breathwork. It begins with simply noticing your breath: its rhythm, its depth, and the sensations as it moves through your body. This quiet act of observation becomes a powerful anchor, grounding you in the present moment and deepening your connection to both body and self.

By turning your attention to your breath, you activate the parasympathetic nervous system—the body's natural calming mechanism. This gentle awareness can reduce stress, regulate the nervous system, and bring clarity to a restless mind. Breath awareness doesn't require effort or control; it's about witnessing rather than managing. Over time, this simple presence cultivates a steadier internal rhythm, helping you meet life's challenges with greater calm, clarity, and resilience.

WHY BREATH AWARENESS IS BENEFICIAL

- Regulates the nervous system
  Tuning into your breath activates the parasympathetic nervous system, shifting you out of "fight-or-flight" and into a state of calm and safety. This supports emotional balance and physical relaxation.

- Increases emotional awareness
  The breath is intimately connected to emotion. Shallow, rapid breaths often accompany anxiety or fear, while deeper, slower breaths reflect calm. By observing your breath, you gain insight into your emotional state and can respond more intentionally.

- Cultivates present-moment awareness
  Your breath is always happening in the now. Focusing on it naturally brings your awareness out of rumination and into the present.

- Supports focus and mental clarity
  Even a few moments of breath awareness can quiet the mind's chatter. This helps improve concentration, sharpen decision-making, and restore perspective.

- Builds the foundation for deeper practices
  Breath awareness is the first step in learning more advanced techniques. It strengthens your capacity for inner attention and prepares you for deeper transformation.

BREATH AWARENESS PRACTICE

1. Find a comfortable position
Sit upright with your spine relaxed, hands resting in your lap or on your knees. You can sit on a chair, cushion, or lie down—whatever feels most supportive.

2. Gently close your eyes
Let your eyelids fall closed to reduce external distractions and bring your focus inward.

3. Notice your breath
Without changing it, bring your attention to your natural breath.

Notice the inhale… and the exhale. Let yourself settle into this rhythm.

4. Tune into sensation
Observe where you feel your breath most clearly—perhaps the nose, chest, or belly. Let your awareness rest there.

5. Allow thoughts to pass
It's natural for thoughts to arise. Gently notice them and return to your breath without judgment.

6. Optional: Lengthen your breath
If it feels right, begin to slowly lengthen each inhale and exhale. Keep it soft and effortless.

7. Stay present
Remain here for a few minutes, simply breathing and noticing.

8. Close gently
When you're ready, open your eyes and take a moment to sense how you feel before continuing your day.

FELT SENSE WITH BODY SCAN

A felt sense refers to the subtle, often unconscious sensations in the body that offer insight into your emotional, mental, and physical state. A body scan is a meditative practice that brings gentle attention to each part of the body, one area at a time.

As you move through this internal landscape, you may notice sensations or areas of tension that were previously hidden. This practice deepens your connection to yourself and offers a bridge between body, mind, and emotion.

WHY FELT SENSE WITH BODY SCAN IS BENEFICIAL

- Increases body awareness
  Develops a deeper sensitivity to your body's signals, helping you notice stress or disconnection before it accumulates.

- Relieves stress and tension
  Consciously softening each part of the body activates the body's natural relaxation response.

- Encourages emotional release
  Tuning into areas of constriction can bring up emotions ready to be acknowledged and released.

- Enhances mindfulness
  Bringing focused attention to each area of the body anchors you in the present moment.

- Cultivates self-compassion
  Listening to your body without judgment fosters trust, care, and acceptance.

FELT SENSE WITH BODY SCAN PRACTICE

1: Find a comfortable position
Sit or lie down in a way that feels fully supported. Close your eyes and take a few slow, grounding breaths.

2: Connect with your breath
Inhale gently through your nose, exhale softly through your mouth. Begin to arrive in your body.

3: Feet
Bring awareness to your feet. Notice any sensations—warmth, pressure, tingling. Breathe into this area.

4: Legs
Move your awareness up through your calves, knees, and thighs. Feel each area and soften as you exhale.

5: Hips and pelvis
Bring gentle attention to your hips and lower back. Breathe into any tension and allow for space.

6: Stomach and abdomen
Notice your belly rising and falling. Let any tightness ease with each breath.

7: Chest and heart space
Bring awareness to your chest, lungs, and heart. Feel expansion on the inhale, softening on the exhale.

8: Shoulders, arms, and hands
Observe this area for tightness or fatigue. Breathe in softness. Release on the exhale.

9: Neck and jaw
Relax the jaw. Let your breath move through the neck and throat. Unclench and allow space.

10: Face and head
Soften the forehead, eyes, scalp. Imagine a gentle wave of ease washing through your head and face.

11: Whole-body awareness
Feel your entire body as a unified whole. Let relaxation ripple through you.

12: End with gratitude
Take a moment to thank your body for its presence, wisdom, and resilience. When you're ready, slowly open your eyes and return to your day.

CHAPTER 19 | BREATHING WITH INTENTION

In the previous chapter, we explored the power of simply noticing—the gentle art of bringing awareness to the breath as it is, and tuning into the felt sense of the body. That foundation of attention prepares us for a subtle shift: from observation to participation.

In this chapter, we begin to work *with* the breath—shaping it, guiding it—with purpose and care. These intentional breathing practices offer a way to influence our internal state, support regulation, and deepen our relationship with breath as an active tool for transformation.

RESISTANCE BREATHING

Resistance breathing involves gently restricting airflow during inhalation and exhalation to engage the respiratory system more deeply. By adding subtle resistance to the breath, you activate respiratory muscles, enhance lung function, and build both physical and mental endurance.

WAYS TO PRACTICE RESISTANCE BREATHING

1. Pursed Lip Breathing
   Exhaling through gently pursed lips creates slight resistance, which slows the breath and promotes a full release of carbon dioxide.

2. Nasal Breathing
   Breathing through the nose instead of the mouth narrows the air passage, encouraging slower, more deliberate breathing and improving oxygen absorption.

3. Ujjayi (Ocean Breath)
   With a soft constriction at the back of the throat, this technique creates an audible, wave-like sound. It slows the breath, calms the nervous system, and generates internal warmth—helping regulate energy and sharpen focus.

Though each of these techniques introduces resistance in a slightly different way, all strengthen respiratory muscles, improve breath control, and support emotional regulation.

WHY RESISTANCE BREATHING IS BENEFICIAL

- Improves lung capacity
  Expands respiratory function and promotes more efficient oxygen exchange.

- Strengthens respiratory muscles
  Builds stamina and breath control by engaging the diaphragm and intercostals.

- Enhances oxygenation
  Slows and deepens the breath, supporting energy and balance through improved CO_2 tolerance.

- Supports calm and stress relief
  Activates the parasympathetic nervous system to reduce anxiety and regulate emotions.

- Boosts mental focus
  Increases oxygen to the brain while anchoring attention, quieting mental chatter.

RESISTANCE BREATHING PRACTICE

1: Settle into a comfortable position
Sit upright with your spine relaxed, or lie down if that feels more supportive. Let your body soften. Eyes may be closed or gently focused.

2: Inhale through your nose
Breathe in slowly for 3–4 seconds. Let the breath expand your belly gently.

3: Exhale through pursed lips
Form your lips as if blowing out a candle. Exhale softly for 5–6 seconds, releasing tension with each out-breath.

4: Repeat the cycle
Continue inhaling through your nose and exhaling through pursed lips for 5–10 minutes. Let your breath stay smooth and effortless.

5: Tune into grounded calm
As your breath slows, sense the stability within you. If helpful, silently repeat a word like *soften, release,* or *I am safe* with each exhale.

Optional: Explore variations
Once comfortable, try nasal-only breathing or the Ujjayi breath variation. With Ujjayi, lightly constrict your throat on both inhale and exhale to create a soft "ocean wave" sound. Let this subtle rhythm draw your focus inward.

COHERENCE BREATHING

Coherence breathing (also known as resonant breathing) involves breathing at a steady, slow rhythm—typically around five to six breaths per minute. A common pattern is a 5-second inhale followed by a 5-second exhale.

This rhythmic breathing helps synchronize your breath and heart rate, increasing *heart rate variability (HRV)* and promoting calm, clarity, and emotional balance. When practiced regularly, coherence breathing supports long-term resilience and improved nervous system regulation.

WHY COHERENCE BREATHING IS BENEFICIAL

- Reduces stress and anxiety
  Shifts the body from fight-or-flight into rest-and-digest mode.
- Improves HRV
  Higher heart rate variability is associated with emotional regulation and better physical health.
- Enhances focus and clarity
  Supports cognitive function and improves decision-making.
- Supports emotional resilience
  Helps you stay grounded and centered in moments of stress or overwhelm.
- Promotes physical well-being
  May help lower blood pressure, support digestion, and ease muscle tension.

COHERENCE BREATHING PRACTICE

1: Find a comfortable position
Sit or lie down with your spine relaxed. Eyes may be closed or softly open.

2: Inhale for five seconds
Breathe in through your nose slowly, letting your belly rise.

3: Exhale for five seconds
Release the breath through your nose, matching the quality and pace of your inhale.

4: Continue the rhythm
Repeat this 5-in/5-out rhythm for 5–10 minutes. Allow your body to relax into the pattern.

5: Add heart-centered imagery
Bring attention to your heart space. Imagine a loved one, a peaceful memory, or a feeling of gratitude. Let this feeling grow with each breath.

Optional: Gradually increase the breath count to 6–6 or beyond, as comfort allows.

DIAPHRAGMATIC BREATHING

Diaphragmatic breathing (also called belly breathing) is the practice of consciously engaging the diaphragm to draw deeper, fuller breaths. As you inhale, your belly expands. As you exhale, it gently contracts. This natural, calming breath resets the stress response and restores energy.

Although belly breathing is innate, many of us default to shallow chest breathing due to stress or posture. Relearning this pattern can profoundly impact your nervous system and overall well-being.

WHY DIAPHRAGMATIC BREATHING IS BENEFICIAL

- Reduces stress and anxiety
- Stimulates the vagus nerve to shift you into a relaxed state.
- Improves oxygenation
  Deep, diaphragmatic breaths boost oxygen flow and energy.
- Balances the nervous system
  Promotes regulation and resilience by shifting out of survival mode.
- Enhances digestion
  Massages internal organs and supports gut function.
- Improves posture
  Encourages upright alignment and reduces lower back tension.
- Promotes better sleep
  Helps unwind the body and prepare for restful sleep.
- Supports emotional release
  Creates space to process and release stored emotions.

DIAPHRAGMATIC BREATHING PRACTICE

1: Find a comfortable position
Sit or lie down in a relaxed posture. Rest one hand on your chest and one on your belly.

2: Inhale through your nose
Breathe in slowly. Let your belly expand outward like a balloon. Keep the chest still.

3: Exhale slowly
Let the belly gently fall as you exhale through your nose or mouth.

4: Continue the rhythm
Keep breathing deeply, allowing each inhale to rise from the belly and each exhale to soften you further.

5: Practice regularly
Begin with 5–10 minutes daily. You can build up over time or use this technique whenever you feel overwhelmed.

CHAPTER 20 | MORE MEDICINE

Box breathing, also known as square breathing, is a simple yet powerful technique that involves four equal phases: inhale, hold, exhale, hold. The name "box" refers to the visual image of a square, with each side representing one phase of the breath.

This structured practice creates a steady, rhythmic flow, calming the nervous system, sharpening focus, and bringing mental clarity. It's easy to incorporate into daily life—whether at work, during moments of stress, or before entering a state of mindful presence.

WHY BOX BREATHING IS BENEFICIAL

- Reduces stress and anxiety
- Regulates the nervous system and activates the parasympathetic response, calming both body and mind.
- Improves focus and concentration
  Counting and rhythm foster presence and help break mental scatter.
- Balances the nervous system
  Harmonizes sympathetic and parasympathetic states to restore internal balance.

- Enhances emotional regulation
  Pauses between breaths help you respond thoughtfully, not react impulsively.
- Increases lung capacity
  Strengthens the diaphragm and supports deeper, more efficient breathing.
- Cultivates mindfulness
  Brings your attention fully to the present, grounding you in your body and breath.

BOX BREATHING PRACTICE

1: Find a comfortable position
Sit with your feet grounded and your spine upright, or lie down if you prefer. Let your body soften.

2: Inhale for a count of 4
Breathe in through your nose, expanding your belly.

3: Hold for a count of 4
Pause gently. Relax your body while retaining the breath.

4: Exhale for a count of 4
Release the breath slowly and steadily through your nose or mouth.

5: Hold after the exhale for a count of 4
Rest in the pause. Feel the stillness.

6: Repeat the cycle
Continue for 5–10 minutes. Adjust the counts as needed to match your capacity, keeping the four phases equal.

4-7-8 BREATHING

The 4-7-8 breath, also called the *relaxing breath*, is a gentle technique designed to reduce stress and calm the nervous system. Popularized by Dr. Andrew Weil, this pattern includes a four-second inhale, seven-second hold, and eight-second exhale. It's especially useful for winding down and preparing the body for rest.

WHY 4-7-8 BREATHING IS BENEFICIAL

- Promotes deep relaxation
  Longer exhales engage the parasympathetic system and encourage a full-body release.
- Improves sleep quality
  Calms the mind and slows the heart rate, preparing the body for rest.
- Reduces anxiety
  Slows racing thoughts and grounds your awareness in the breath.
- Improves oxygen exchange
  Enhances respiratory function and deepens your breath.
- Supports cardiovascular health
  Lowers blood pressure and heart rate by regulating stress responses.
- Encourages mindfulness
  The rhythmic count helps anchor you in the present.

4-7-8 BREATHING PRACTICE

1: Find a comfortable position
Sit or lie down with your spine relaxed. Close your eyes if it feels supportive.

2: Inhale for 4 seconds
Breathe in gently through your nose, allowing your belly to expand.

3: Hold for 7 seconds
Retain the breath calmly. Let the stillness be spacious, not tense.

4: Exhale for 8 seconds
Release the breath through your nose or mouth. Let the breath fall away like a slow sigh.

5: Repeat
Continue for 4–8 cycles. With practice, you may extend to several minutes, especially before bed or during moments of overwhelm.

ALTERNATE NOSTRIL BREATHING

Alternate nostril breathing (or "Nadi Shodhana") is a traditional yogic practice that balances energy, harmonizes the brain hemispheres, and calms the nervous system. "nadi" means channel or energy pathway, and "shodhana" means purification. This technique clears blockages in the energetic body, allowing prana (life force) to move freely.

By alternating nostrils with each breath, you create internal balance, quiet the mind, and prepare the body for deeper states of peace or meditation.

WHY ALTERNATE NOSTRIL BREATHING IS BENEFICIAL

- Balances the nervous system
  Harmonizes sympathetic and parasympathetic activity for equilibrium.

- Reduces stress and anxiety
  Slows the breath and stills the mind.

- Improves mental clarity and focus
  Increases oxygen to the brain and strengthens attention.

- Balances brain hemispheres
  Left nostril activates calm; right nostril boosts energy. Alternating promotes integration.

- Supports emotional stability
  Brings calm presence and smooths emotional highs and lows.

- Prepares for meditation
  Calms the body and mind, deepening awareness.

ALTERNATE NOSTRIL BREATHING PRACTICE

1: Sit comfortably
Sit cross-legged or in a chair with your spine tall. Rest your left hand in your lap.

2: Prepare your right hand
Place your right thumb near your right nostril and your ring finger near your left. Your index and middle fingers can rest on your forehead.

3: Inhale through the left nostril
Close your right nostril with your thumb. Inhale slowly through your left nostril.

4: Close the left, exhale through the right
Use your ring finger to close the left nostril. Release your thumb and exhale through the right.

5: Inhale through the right nostril
Breathe in gently through the right side.

6: Close the right, exhale through the left
Close the right nostril and exhale through the left.

7: Repeat
This is one full cycle. Continue for 5–10 rounds, moving with steady rhythm and relaxed awareness.

BREATH HOLDING

Breath retention (or "*Kumbhaka*" in yogic terms) involves pausing after the inhale or exhale. This practice builds internal awareness, strengthens the respiratory system, and increases emotional resilience. It's not about forcing or holding until discomfort—but about creating conscious space in the breath.

Why Breath Holding Is Beneficial

- Improves oxygen efficiency
  Trains the body to use oxygen more effectively and builds endurance.
- Stimulates the parasympathetic nervous system
  Encourages rest and recovery through the pause.
- Enhances CO_2 tolerance
  Builds calm resilience in the face of rising CO_2—especially useful for anxiety and breathlessness.
- Increases mental clarity and focus
  The pause between breaths invites stillness and presence.
- Stimulates the vagus nerve
  Improves vagal tone and stress response regulation.
- Promotes emotional resilience
  Teaches how to be with discomfort, building capacity for inner stillness and steadiness.

BREATH HOLDING PRACTICE

1: Get comfortable
Sit or lie down with your spine aligned. Close your eyes and take a few natural breaths.

2: Inhale slowly
Breathe in through your nose for 4–5 seconds, filling your lungs.

3: Hold the breath
Pause at the top of the inhale for 4–7 seconds. Stay soft and relaxed.

4: Exhale slowly
Release the breath through your nose or mouth for 6–8 seconds.

5: Hold after the exhale
Pause at the bottom of the breath for 3–5 seconds.

6: Repeat the cycle
Continue for 5–10 rounds, or as feels supportive. Afterward, sit quietly and notice how you feel.

CHAPTER 21 | BREATHING FOR EMOTIONAL RELEASE

As we begin to work with the breath more intentionally, we open the door not only to regulation—but to *release*. Breath has a way of reaching into places words often can't: deep into the tissues, the nervous system, the hidden corners where emotion is held.

This chapter explores how specific breath practices can support the safe expression and softening of stored emotions, offering a pathway to clarity, lightness, and healing from within.

BREATH OF FIRE

Breath of Fire is a rapid, rhythmic breath technique involving quick, forceful exhales through the nose, while allowing the inhale to occur passively. Often called "the breath of transformation," it's known for awakening energy, igniting inner fire (*agni*), and stimulating detoxification. Common in Kundalini yoga, this breath also strengthens the diaphragm and core, clears the mind, and boosts vitality.

WHY BREATH OF FIRE IS BENEFICIAL

- Energizes the body
  Stimulates oxygen intake, clears mental fog, and offers an instant energy lift.
- Detoxifies the system
  Promotes circulation and lymphatic flow to release waste and support internal cleansing.
- Stimulates digestion
  Massages abdominal organs and enhances *agni*, reducing bloating and improving gut health.
- Balances the nervous system
  Engages both sympathetic and parasympathetic activity for clarity and calm.
- Strengthens diaphragm and core
  Builds respiratory strength, increases lung capacity, and tones abdominal muscles.
- Regulates emotions
  Releases emotional tension, especially anger or frustration, and supports emotional resilience.

BREATH OF FIRE PRACTICE

1: Find a comfortable seat
Sit cross-legged or on a chair with your spine tall and shoulders relaxed.

2: Relax and prepare
Take a few deep breaths to settle. Soften your face, jaw, and eyes.

3: Begin with exhalation
Inhale naturally, then sharply exhale through the nose. Your belly will naturally draw in; the inhale is passive.

4: Establish a rhythmic pace
Start at 2–3 breaths per second. Practice for 15–30 seconds, gradually increasing to 1–3 minutes as comfortable.

5: Engage your core
Let the exhale originate from your diaphragm. Feel your belly actively contract.

6: Focus your awareness
Stay with the breath. If the mind wanders, return to the rhythm—or optionally add a silent mantra.

7: Close slowly
When ready, slow the breath. Sit quietly and observe any energetic or emotional shifts.

CONSCIOUS CONNECTED BREATHING

Conscious Connected Breathing is a continuous, flowing pattern of breath without pauses between inhale and exhale. This uninterrupted rhythm encourages the free movement of energy and emotion through the body, often resulting in deep release and clarity.

This practice is especially powerful for emotional processing, nervous system healing, and reconnecting with your body's innate wisdom.

WHY CONSCIOUS CONNECTED BREATHING IS BENEFICIAL

- Facilitates emotional release
  Surfaces and softens stored emotions, supporting gentle expression and healing.

- Clears energetic blockages
  Moves stagnant energy and restores vitality throughout the body's energetic systems.

- Increases oxygen and energy flow
  Boosts oxygenation and cellular function while awakening natural vitality.

- Promotes relaxation and stress relief
  Regulates the nervous system and creates a calming rhythm of breath.

- Enhances mental clarity
  Sharpens presence, deepens awareness, and improves decision-making.

- Strengthens mind-body connection
  Cultivates embodied awareness, intuition, and self-trust.

- Supports personal growth
  Unveils limiting patterns and beliefs, offering a pathway to transformation.

CONSCIOUS CONNECTED BREATHING PRACTICE

1: Find a comfortable position
Sit or lie down in a safe, quiet space. Keep your spine relaxed and body supported.

2: Begin with gentle breaths
Inhale through your nose and exhale through your mouth. Let your breath begin to settle.

3: Establish the circular breath
Inhale deeply through the mouth, then exhale without pause. The inhale is active, the exhale passive. Each breath flows into the next with no gaps. (Nasal breathing is also okay if preferred.)

4: Stay present
Notice sensations. Emotions or tension may arise—stay with the breath and allow release.

5: Extend the practice gradually
Start with 5–10 minutes and build toward 30+ minutes over time. Let the breath deepen naturally.

6: Close with stillness
After the last breath, lie quietly. Notice any feelings of openness, energy, or peace. Gently return to your day.

LION'S BREATH

Lion's Breath is a bold and expressive technique involving a strong exhale through the mouth while sticking out the tongue. Often used to release tension, clear frustration, or boost confidence, this breath invites playfulness, power, and embodied freedom.

It's especially helpful for emotional stagnation or when you need to shake off heaviness and reconnect with your strength.

WHY LION'S BREATH IS BENEFICIAL

- Releases tension
  Clears stress from the jaw, face, and neck—common areas for stored tension.
- Improves mental clarity
  Cuts through fog and encourages full-body presence.
- Energizes and uplifts
  Stimulates parasympathetic response while offering a natural energy boost.
- Fosters emotional expression
  Provides a safe outlet for anger, stress, or unspoken feelings.
- Activates the throat and heart chakras
  Supports clear communication, courage, and emotional balance.
- Promotes confidence
  Breaks through inhibition and supports empowered, authentic expression.

LION'S BREATH PRACTICE

1: Find a seated posture
Sit tall, with hands resting on your knees. Spread your fingers wide.

2: Take a deep inhale
Breathe in through your nose, filling your lungs fully.

3: Exhale with a roar
Open your mouth wide, stick out your tongue, and exhale forcefully. Make a sound if it feels good—like a roar or release.

4: Focus on the release
Visualize letting go of tension, emotion, or stress as the breath leaves your body.

5: Repeat 5–10 rounds
Pause between rounds to feel any shifts. Let yourself be playful or fierce.

6: Close in stillness
After your final round, sit quietly and breathe normally. Feel the afterglow of release and strength.

INTEGRATION | THE BREATH WITHIN AND THROUGHOUT

As we close this section of breathwork exploration, this isn't about discovering something new—it's about deepening into what's already within you. What's always been here, waiting for your attention.

The breath has been both your tool and your teacher. It has guided you into stillness, clarity, and release. It has asked you to trust the pauses, expand your presence, and loosen your grip.

But the breath does not stand alone. It moves through everything you've been nurturing: your inner awareness, your capacity to feel, your body, your voice, your connection to others. Integration is where transformation shifts from knowing to living—where practice becomes presence.

This is your invitation: not to strive, but to return—with gentleness and curiosity.

Let your breath meet your mind, body and heart.
Let it shape the sacred ordinary of your life.

CONCLUSION | COMING HOME

If you've made it this far, I honor the quiet courage that brought you here. The willingness to read, to feel, to stay—these are acts of transformation. Whether you've breathed with me through every page or simply allowed yourself to be seen in parts, you've already begun.

Healing is rarely linear. Some days feel ordinary. Others bring breakthroughs. Both are sacred. The key is not to rush, not to perfect, but to stay present—to keep choosing yourself again and again.

A WAY OF LIVING

The Lifelines—Radical Self-Love, Feel All Your Feelings, Bend, Breathe, Sound, Circle, Express, Heart & Hands, and Body Temple—are not a checklist. They are a way of living, a scaffolding for your life. They anchor you in presence, invite awareness, and remind you of the wholeness that's always been yours.

Start with one. Practice it. Let it integrate. When it feels right, weave in another. Each ritual—whether a deep breath, a stretch, a hand on your heart, a kind word, or a creative expression—is a gentle act of self-remembrance. Over time, these small, ordinary practices compound, creating a quiet, steady foundation for your resilience, clarity, and joy.

RECLAIMING YOUR VOICE

This journey isn't about perfection. It's about honoring your story—every part of it. Even the pieces you were told to hide.

When you accept your past without shame, you free yourself. When you reclaim your voice, you reclaim your power. You no longer need permission to exist fully, to speak your truth, to hold your boundaries. Sovereignty begins not when the world believes you, but when you believe yourself.

Through Breath, Circle, and Express, I found the courage to speak, to listen, and to hold space for my own heart—and for others. These practices are both compass and anchor, helping you navigate storms without losing sight of your center.

FROM PAIN TO PURPOSE

This book was born from loss, but also from quiet rebellion—the decision to stop performing, stop proving, and start remembering. Breathwork found me not as a trend, but as a necessity. Through it, I began reclaiming my body, my presence, and my power. From that reclamation, I could hold space for others to do the same.

Letting go of external expectations and systems that no longer served me was not easy. But in that letting go, I discovered a profound beginning: the power to live from choice, from love, from presence.

THIS IS WHAT COMES NEXT

In your own life, the steps forward may feel small. But they matter. Solitude can be a reckoning, reflection a guide. Breath becomes a threshold—an ever-available tool to anchor, release, and return.

You are no longer defined by what happened. You are defined by the life you choose to create.

You choose to breathe.

To stay.

To feel.

To rise.

And when you forget—when fear creeps in or the world feels too loud—you come back to your breath.

Again and again, as many times as it takes.

CLOSING RITUAL

Before you move into your daily life, pause.
Which Lifeline calls to you most today?
What small act of presence, care, or expression could you honor right now?

Let it be small. Let it be real. Healing doesn't have to be dramatic. Often, it's found in the softest places: a glass of water, a breath, a truth spoken aloud. What matters is not how perfectly you practice—but that you begin.

CLOSING BREATH PRACTICE:

1. Settle In
   Find a quiet space. Sit or lie down. One hand on your heart, one on your belly. Let your body be held.

2. Grounding Inhale
   Inhale through your nose for 4
   Hold for 2
   Exhale through your mouth for 6
   Soften your shoulders. Release your jaw.

3. Integration
   Inhale: *I belong to myself*
   Exhale: *I am free*
   Repeat for several rounds.

4. Closing
   Place both hands on your heart. Take one final, steady breath. Feel the truth of your becoming. You are home.

CLOSING AFFIRMATIONS:

I trust the truth of my experience.

I am the author of my healing and the keeper of my worth.

I reclaim my breath, my body, and my becoming.

I choose presence, sovereignty, and love—again and again.

EPILOGUE | A FINAL NOTE ON SOVEREIGNTY (AND WHAT COMES NEXT)

As I finish this book—three years after the assault and arrest—my legal battle is finally coming to a close. I chose not to recount every detail here, but I will say this: the resistance I faced was deeply unjust. And yet, it shaped something unshakable in me.

The more I was questioned, dismissed, or betrayed, the more deeply I rooted into my own knowing—not just about what happened, but about who I am.

Some of the most painful wounds came not from institutions, but from people I once trusted. But that rupture created a clarity I had never known. I stopped trying to prove I was good, worthy, or believable. I simply began to trust myself—and to know, *that is enough.*

That same clarity asked me to face a question I still carry:

How do we hold both the fire to speak and the tenderness to lead from our hearts?

When injustice strips us of power, there is a pull toward constant opposition, constant proving. Rage, when denied, festers. But, when wielded with care, it can become a compass. And yet living in that stance alone can become toxic and exhausting.

I am learning that sovereignty is the meeting place of both—the part of me that refuses to shrink and the part of me that knows when to release the fight.

I can advocate without carrying every burden.
I can use my voice without letting the mission consume my breath.
I can meet opposition without becoming it.

This is not an ending; it is a threshold. I can return to myself again and again, grounded, steady, whole—and so can you. Pause. Breathe. Feel. You are already home.

*"When we meet the breaking with breath,
we begin to uncover the gold within the wreckage."*

— Romy Limenes

AFTERWORD | A CALL FOR CHANGE

While this book has been a personal journey, it points to something much larger. Healing is never isolated. Personal transformation is tied to collective responsibility.

If you or someone you love has experienced being drugged without consent, please hear this clearly:
It is not your fault.
You deserve to be believed. You deserve safety. You deserve support.

My story revealed painful gaps in the very systems meant to protect us.
This is not just personal—it's systemic. It's public. And it calls for change.

We need:

- Standardized and mandated drug screening protocols in hospitals, jails, and by first responders—so that involuntary or non-consensual drug intoxication can be detected early, documented, and treated appropriately.

- Legislation requiring businesses that serve alcohol to have video surveillance in all customer areas, with a mandated retention period. This would preserve evidence if a patron was drugged or assaulted and help deter misconduct by staff or others."

- Trauma- and drug-assault-informed training for healthcare providers, police officers, correctional staff, EMTs, and crisis responders—ensuring they understand the physical, psychological, and behavioral signs of drug-facilitated assault, including memory loss, confusion, difficulty speaking or standing, emotional volatility, signs of nervous system overwhelm, and nausea with or without vomiting.

- Clear procedures and accountability for collecting and preserving evidence in suspected cases of drug-facilitated assault—even when a person is disoriented, unable to give consent in the moment, or struggling to recall what happened. This should include the timely use of a sexual assault forensic exam (rape kit), as sexual violence may have occurred without the individual's awareness."

- Legislation that expands definitions of assault to include drug-facilitated harm, improves access to justice, and mandates investigation even when traditional evidence is limited.

- Cross-agency collaboration between medical professionals, law enforcement, forensic labs, and advocacy groups to improve survivor outcomes and eliminate systemic negligence.

- A cultural shift—one that replaces blame with belief, skepticism with compassion, and silence with systemic awareness. Survivors deserve to be met with care, not criminalization.

Until our systems evolve to recognize and respond to the reality of drug-facilitated assault, we will continue to retraumatize the very people we are meant to protect.

For too long, silence has protected systems—not survivors. That must change.

Here's how you can help:

- Call your local representatives. Demand better protections and protocols.
- Support survivor-led organizations and advocacy work.
- Speak out—share your story, or help amplify someone else's.
- Listen without judgment. Believe survivors.
- Create spaces of safety, care, and respect in your communities.

Every voice matters.

Every action counts.

Together, we can build a world where survivors are supported, not silenced.

STAY CONNECTED WITH ME

Though this book is ending, our connection doesn't have to.

Whether you're brand new to breathwork or have been walking this path for years, I hope something in these pages brought you a moment of presence, a breath of relief, or a reminder of your inner strength.

If this work has resonated with you, I'd love to stay connected. I offer live classes, personalized guided sessions, and private coaching for those ready to delve deeper.

With gratitude, breath and strength,

Romy

ABOUT THE AUTHOR

Romy Limenes is a breathwork facilitator and trauma-informed coach devoted to helping others reclaim their calm, their clarity, and their inner power—one breath at a time. Her work lives at the intersection of simplicity and healing, offering gentle, embodied practices for nervous system regulation, resilience, and reconnection.

Before stepping into this work, Romy spent over two decades as a registered nurse, supporting others through the physical and emotional terrain of healing. That experience continues to inform her grounded, heart-led approach.

A mother, a survivor, and a steady guide, Romy teaches from lived experience—with softness, truth, and quiet strength. She is the founder of Breathwork Simple, where she offers live classes, coaching, and a growing body of resources designed to help others return to themselves.

Broken to Breathful is her first book.

You can find Romy and explore her other offerings and resources at breathworksimple.com and on Instagram @romylimenes.

ROMY'S FAVORITE READS

These books have been my companions—through seasons of transformation, moments of stillness, and years of deep inquiry. Each one has offered me insight, comfort, or a nudge toward growth. Whether you're new to the path or well on your way, I hope you'll find something here that resonates with your journey.

BREATH & EMBODIMENT

Breath: The New Science of a Lost Art by James Nestor
A compelling exploration into the forgotten science of breathing. This book reignited my respect for the simple, vital act of breath and its profound role in health and well-being.

Just Breathe: Mastering Breathwork by Dan Brulé
A practical and inspiring guide to breathwork techniques from a seasoned teacher. This book helped bridge the gap between science and spirituality for me.

The Healing Power of the Breath by Richard P. Brown & Patricia L. Gerbarg
Grounded in both modern psychiatry and ancient practices, this book gave me practical tools to regulate anxiety and emotional overwhelm through the breath.

Feel to Heal: Releasing Trauma Through Body Awareness and Breathwork by Giten Tonkov
A deeply somatic approach to emotional healing through breath. This book affirmed much of what I've experienced in my own work and added nuance to my understanding of trauma and the body.

TRAUMA, NERVOUS SYSTEM & SOMATIC HEALING

Waking the Tiger: Healing Trauma by Peter Levine
One of the foundational texts on somatic experiencing. Levine's work opened my eyes to how trauma lives in the body—and how it can be released.

The Body Keeps the Score: Brain, Mind, and Body in the Healing of Trauma by Bessel van der Kolk
A cornerstone in trauma literature. This book helped me contextualize so much of what I've felt but couldn't name.

The Tao of Fully Feeling: Harvesting Forgiveness Out of Blame by Pete Walker
Compassionate and raw, this book helped me navigate emotional wounding and the path to forgiveness—of self and others.

RELATIONSHIPS & EMOTIONAL COMMUNICATION

Conscious Loving by Gay and Kathlyn Hendricks
A game-changer in the way I show up in relationships. It taught me that deep love requires deep honesty and presence.

Relationships That Work: The Power of Conscious Living by David B. Wolf
A powerful guide to bringing mindfulness and integrity into all of our relationships.

Nonviolent Communication: A Language of Life by Marshall B. Rosenberg
A practical roadmap for speaking and listening from the heart.

This book changed the way I engage in conflict and cultivate empathy.

SPIRITUAL GROUNDING & PRESENCE

The Power of Now by Eckhart Tolle
The first book that truly taught me the value of the present moment. It marked a turning point in my inner life.

Loving What Is: Four Questions That Can Change Your Life by Byron Katie
A deceptively simple process that softened much of my inner resistance. A reminder that peace often comes from perspective.

Fear: Essential Wisdom for Getting Through the Storm by Thich Nhat Hanh
Gentle and wise, this book taught me how to sit with fear instead of pushing it away.

Welcoming the Unwelcome: Wholehearted Living in a Brokenhearted World by Pema Chödrön
This book reminded me that there is no spiritual bypassing. Healing requires us to face life with an open heart—even when it breaks.

The Five Invitations: Discovering What Death Can Teach Us About Living Fully by Frank Ostaseski
A profoundly moving reflection on impermanence. This book shaped how I approach life, love, and breath—with deeper reverence.

COMPASSION, RESILIENCE & PERSONAL GROWTH

Tattoos on the Heart: The Power of Boundless Compassion by Gregory Boyle
A collection of stories that broke me open and stitched me back together. A masterclass in love without judgment.

The Gifts of Imperfection by Brené Brown
A rally cry for authenticity and self-acceptance. This book helped me lean into vulnerability, one small act at a time.

Love Warrior by Glennon Doyle
Raw, unfiltered, and brave. Doyle's honesty about pain and transformation mirrored much of my own journey.

The Let Them Theory by Mel Robbins
A refreshing and liberating perspective on letting go of control and people-pleasing.

30 Days to a New Relationship with Alcohol by Holly Whitaker
A beautiful, raw, and no-nonsense tribute to any woman on a journey of self-reclamation and radical self-love. This book reminds us again and again that we are exactly where we're meant to be.

Help, Thanks, Wow: The Three Essential Prayers by Anne Lamott
A small but mighty book. Lamott reminds us that spiritual practice doesn't have to be complicated—it can begin with just a few honest words.

You Are the Placebo by Dr. Joe Dispenza
This book opened my eyes to the mind's influence over the body. A profound reminder that belief, intention, and breath are powerful agents of change.

REFERENCES

FOUNDATIONAL BREATHWORK & PHYSIOLOGY

Zaccaro, A., et al. (2018). How breath-control can change your life: A systematic review on psycho-physiological correlates of slow breathing. Frontiers in Human Neuroscience.

Lehrer, P. M., Eddie, D., & Yeh, G. (2020). Resonance frequency breathing: Theoretical foundations and clinical applications. International Journal of Psychophysiology.

Lehrer, P. M., et al. (2000). Heart rate variability biofeedback increases baroreflex gain and peak expiratory flow. Applied Psychophysiology and Biofeedback.

Brown, R. P., & Gerbarg, P. L. (2005). Sudarshan Kriya yogic breathing in the treatment of stress, anxiety, and depression. Journal of Alternative and Complementary Medicine.

Jerath, R., et al. (2006). Physiology of long pranayamic breathing. Medical Hypotheses.

Noble, D. J., & Hochman, S. (2019). Pulmonary afferent activity and relaxation. Frontiers in Physiology.

Van Diest, I., et al. (2001). Hyperventilation and the Bohr effect. Clinical Physiology.

Nestor, J. (2020). Breath: The New Science of a Lost Art. Riverhead Books.

Gerbarg, P. L., & Brown, R. P. (2012). The Healing Power of the Breath. Shambhala Publications.

TRAUMA & SOMATIC HEALING

Van der Kolk, B. A. (2014). The Body Keeps the Score: Brain, Mind, and Body in the Healing of Trauma. Viking.

Levine, P. A. (2010). In an Unspoken Voice: How the Body Releases Trauma and Restores Goodness. North Atlantic Books.

Levine, P. A. (1997). Waking the Tiger: Healing Trauma. North Atlantic Books.

Ogden, P., & Fisher, J. (2015). Sensorimotor Psychotherapy: Interventions for Trauma and Attachment. W. W. Norton.

Ogden, P., Minton, K., & Pain, C. (2006). Trauma and the Body: A Sensorimotor Approach to Psychotherapy. W. W. Norton.

Rothschild, B. (2000). The Body Remembers: The Psychophysiology of Trauma and Trauma Treatment. W. W. Norton.

Emerson, D., & Hopper, E. (2011). Overcoming Trauma Through Yoga: Reclaiming Your Body. North Atlantic Books.

Tonkov, G. (2021). Feel to Heal: Releasing Trauma Through Body Awareness and Breathwork. Breathwork Academy.

Maté, G. (2003). When the Body Says No: Exploring the Stress-Disease Connection. Wiley.

POLYVAGAL THEORY & NERVOUS SYSTEM REGULATION

Porges, S. W. (2011). The Polyvagal Theory: Neurophysiological Foundations of Emotions, Attachment, Communication, and Self-Regulation. W. W. Norton.

Porges, S. W. (2017). The Pocket Guide to Polyvagal Theory: The Transformative Power of Feeling Safe. W. W. Norton.

Tracey, K. J. (2007). Physiology and immunology of the cholinergic anti-inflammatory pathway. The Journal of Clinical Investigation.

INTEROCEPTION, MINDFULNESS & BODY AWARENESS

Mehling, W. E., et al. (2012). The Multidimensional Assessment of Interoceptive Awareness (MAIA). PLOS ONE.

Mehling, W. E., et al. (2012). Body awareness in mind-body therapies: Contributions to research and practice.Philosophy, Ethics, and Humanities in Medicine.

Hölzel, B. K., et al. (2011). How does mindfulness meditation work? Proposing mechanisms of action from a conceptual and neural perspective. Perspectives on Psychological Science.

Siegel, D. J. (2010). The Mindful Therapist: A Clinician's Guide to Mindsight and Neural Integration. W. W. Norton.

Kabat-Zinn, J. (2005). Wherever You Go, There You Are: Mindfulness Meditation in Everyday Life. Hachette Books.

EMOTIONAL HEALING, SELF-COMPASSION & RESILIENCE

Neff, K. (2011). Self-Compassion: The Proven Power of Being Kind to Yourself. William Morrow.

Brown, B. (2010). The Gifts of Imperfection: Let Go of Who You Think You're Supposed to Be and Embrace Who You Are. Hazelden Publishing.

Brown, B. (2018). Braving the Wilderness: The Quest for True Belonging and the Courage to Stand Alone. Random House.

Robbins, M. (2023). The Let Them Theory. [Self-published.]

Linehan, M. M. (1993). Cognitive-Behavioral Treatment of Borderline Personality Disorder. Guilford Press.

Hanson, R. (2013). Hardwiring Happiness: The New Brain Science of Contentment, Calm, and Confidence. Harmony Books.

Gendlin, E. T. (1981). Focusing. Bantam Books.

DeSteno, D. (2018). Emotional Success: The Power of Gratitude, Compassion, and Pride. Eamon Dolan/Houghton Mifflin Harcourt.

STRESS, EXERCISE & HEALTH

Sapolsky, R. M. (2004). Why Zebras Don't Get Ulcers: The Acclaimed Guide to Stress, Stress-Related Diseases, and Coping. Holt Paperbacks.

Ratey, J. J. (2008). Spark: The Revolutionary New Science of Exercise and the Brain. Little, Brown.

Erickson, K. I., et al. (2011). Exercise training increases size of hippocampus and improves memory. Proceedings of the National Academy of Sciences (PNAS).

Harvard Health Publishing. (2020). Exercising to relax. Harvard Medical School.

Popkin, B. M., et al. (2010). Water, hydration, and health. Nutrition Reviews.

Walker, M. (2017). Why We Sleep: Unlocking the Power of Sleep and Dreams. Scribner.

COMMUNITY, CONNECTION & OXYTOCIN

Carter, C. S. (2014). Oxytocin pathways and the evolution of human behavior. Annual Review of Psychology.

Heinrichs, M., et al. (2003). Social support and oxytocin interact to suppress cortisol and subjective responses to psychosocial stress. Biological Psychiatry.

House, J. S., et al. (1988). Social relationships and health. Science.

Umberson, D., & Montez, J. K. (2010). Social relationships and health: A flashpoint for health policy. Journal of Health and Social Behavior.

Holt-Lunstad, J., et al. (2010). Social relationships and mortality risk: A meta-analytic review. PLOS Medicine.

Baumeister, R. F., & Leary, M. R. (1995). The need to belong: Desire for interpersonal attachments as a fundamental human motivation. Psychological Bulletin.

Seppälä, E. (2016). The Happiness Track: How to Apply the Science of Happiness to Accelerate Your Success. HarperOne.

Siegel, D. J. (2012). The Developing Mind: How Relationships and the Brain Interact to Shape Who We Are. Guilford Press.

SOUND HEALING, FLOW & CREATIVITY

Goldsby, T. L., et al. (2017). Effects of singing bowl sound meditation on mood, tension, and well-being: An observational study. Journal of Evidence-Based Integrative Medicine.

Le Scouarnec, R. P., et al. (2001). Binaural beat tapes for anxiety: A pilot study. Alternative Therapies.

Mason, J. S., & Brady, K. (2007). Brainwave entrainment and binaural beats: Cognitive and emotional effects. Cognitive Neuroscience Journal.

Austin, D. (2008). The Theory and Practice of Vocal Psychotherapy: Songs of the Self. Jessica Kingsley.

Dietrich, A. (2004). Neurocognitive mechanisms of flow. Consciousness and Cognition.

Levitin, D. J. (2019). This Is Your Brain on Music: The Science of a Human Obsession. Dutton.

Forgeard, M. J. C., & Elstein, J. G. (2014). Advancing the clinical science of creativity. Frontiers in Psychology.

King, L. A. (2001). Health benefits of writing about life goals. Personality and Social Psychology Bulletin.

Ulrich, R. S. (1984). View through a window may influence recovery from surgery. Science.

Stuckey, H. L., & Nobel, J. (2010). Art, healing, and public health: A review of current literature. American Journal of Public Health.

POSITIVE PSYCHOLOGY, GRATITUDE & MINDSET

Crum, A. J., et al. (2013). Rethinking stress: The role of mindsets. Journal of Personality and Social Psychology.

Emmons, R. A., & McCullough, M. E. (2003). Counting blessings versus burdens: An experimental investigation of gratitude and subjective well-being in daily life. Journal of Personality and Social Psychology.

McGonigal, K. (2015). The Upside of Stress: Why Stress Is Good for You, and How to Get Good at It. Avery.

Huberman, A. (2023). Tools for calming the nervous system. The Huberman Lab Podcast. [Referenced in educational materials.]

www.ingramcontent.com/pod-product-compliance
Lightning Source LLC
LaVergne TN
LVHW020931090426
835512LV00020B/3311